EXERCISE AND MENTAL HEALTH

The Series in Health Psychology and Behavioral Medicine

Charles D. Spielberger, *Editor-in-Chief*

Chesney, Rosenman Anger and Hostility in Cardiovascular
  and Behavioral Disorders
Lonetto, Templer Death Anxiety
Morgan, Goldston Exercise and Mental Health

IN PREPARATION

Elias, Marshall Cardiovascular Disease and Behavior
Hobfoll Ecology of Stress
Pancheri, Zichelli Biorhythms and Stress in the Physiopathology
  of Reproduction

EXERCISE
AND MENTAL HEALTH

Edited by

WILLIAM P. MORGAN
University of Wisconsin–Madison

STEPHEN E. GOLDSTON
University of California at Los Angeles

● HEMISPHERE PUBLISHING CORPORATION
A member of the Taylor & Francis Group

New York   Washington   Philadelphia   London

EXERCISE AND MENTAL HEALTH

3 4 5 6 7 8 9 BCBC 8 9 8

This book was set in Times Roman by Hemisphere Publishing Corporation. The editors were Christine Flint Lowry and Eleana Cornejo-de-Villanueva; the production supervisor was Peggy M. Rote; and the typesetter was Cynthia B. Mynhier.
BookCrafters, Inc. was printer and binder.

Library of Congress Cataloging in Publication Data

Exercise and mental health.

   (The Series in health psychology and behavioral medicine)
   Includes bibliographies and index.
   1. Mental health.   2. Exercise therapy.   3. Mental
illness—Prevention.   4. Stress (Psychology)—Prevention.
I. Morgan, William P.   II. Goldston, Stephen E.
III. Series. [DNLM: 1. Exercise Therapy.   2. Exertion
3. Mental Disorders—therapy.   4. Physical Fitness.
WM 405 E96]
RA790.E94   1987   616.89′13   86-14817
ISBN 0-89116-564-9
ISSN 8756-467X

TO THE MEMORY OF

Professor A. H. Ismail

Athlete, scientist, transcendentalist, and pioneer in the investigation of mechanisms underlying the relationship between exercise and mental health.

CONTENTS

Chapter 5

Chapter 6

Part III PREVENTION AND TREATMENT

Chapter 7

CONTRIBUTORS

Bonnie G. Berger, Ed.D., Professor and Director, Sport Psychology Laboratory, Brooklyn College of the City University of New York.

Robert S. Brown, M.D., Ph.D., Clinical Associate Professor, Department of Behavioral Medicine and Psychiatry, University of Virginia Medical School and Professor of Education, Department of Educational Foundations, University of Virginia.

Herbert A. deVries, Ph.D., F.A.C.S.M., Emeritus Professor of Physical Education, University of Southern California and Director, Mobile Electromyography Laboratory, South Laguna, CA.

Rod K. Dishman, Ph.D., F.A.C.S.M., Associate Professor, Department of Physical Education, University of Georgia.

Stephen E. Goldston, Ed.D., M.S.P.H., Consultant in Preventive Psychiatry, The Neuropsychiatric Institute, University of California at Los Angeles, and Former Director, Office of Prevention, National Institute of Mental Health.

John H. Greist, M.D., Professor, Department of Psychiatry, University of Wisconsin-Madison.

Dorothy V. Harris, Ph.D., F.A.C.S.M., Professor and Director, Center for Women in Sports, Pennsylvania State University.

William L. Haskell, Ph.D., F.A.C.S.M., Clinical Associate Professor of Medicine, Stanford University Medical Center, Stanford Heart Disease Prevention Program.

A. H. Ismail, H.S.D. (Deceased), Late Professor, Department of Physical Education, Purdue University.

Daniel S. Kirschenbaum, Ph.D., Department of Psychiatry, Northwestern University Medical School.

Egil W. Martinsen, M.D., Psychiatrist, Modum Bads Nervesanatorium, Norway.

William P. Morgan, Ed.D., F.A.C.S.M., Professor and Director, Sport Psychology Laboratory, University of Wisconsin-Madison.

Michael L. Sachs, Ph.D., Research Project Coordinator, Adult Services-DD Program, University of Maryland School of Medicine, Baltimore.

Wesley E. Sime, Ph.D., M.P.H., Associate Professor and Director, Stress Physiology Laboratory, University of Nebraska-Lincoln.

Charles D. Spielberger, Ph.D., Professor of Psychology and Director, Center for Research in Behavioral Medicine and Community Psychology, University of South Florida, Tampa.

PREFACE

Exercise has been advocated by health scientists and physicians for many years as a means of preventing physical health problems, such as obesity and hypertension. Its efficacy as a therapeutic measure once certain illnesses have occurred has been extolled as well. Although exercise enthusiasts have acknowledged the absence of compelling empirical evidence to support such views, they have maintained that regular exercise has intuitive appeal. The past decade has witnessed the emergence of the view that exercise also can prevent the onset of emotional problems. Furthermore, many health professionals now believe that vigorous exercise is an effective treatment once mental health problems develop. For example, a survey in 1983 of nearly 2000 primary-care physicians revealed that 85 percent regularly prescribed exercise in the treatment of depression.

Given the pandemic nature of such mental health problems as anxiety and depression—in concert with the cost and time associated with traditional psychotherapy, as well as the cost and potential side- or after-effects of various drugs used in the treatment of these problems—it would seem important to quantify the efficacy of exercise as a coping strategy. Indeed, if exercise were found to be effective in the primary and secondary prevention of mental health problems, and if there were no significant after- or side-effects, exercise would hold the potential for becoming the treatment of choice. Unfortunately, no effort has been forthcoming to consolidate existing knowledge on this topic—at least not in a scientifically defensible context.

This volume has been developed in an effort to present a state-of-the-art summary of what is known about exercise and mental health. It is hoped that such information will be of direct value to psychologists, physicians, physical educators, and exercise leaders concerned with both the preservation and restoration of health in their students, clients, and patients. We believe this volume can serve as a desk reference for health professionals interested in using exercise in primary and secondary prevention efforts. The book also addresses the psychobiological impact of exercise on individuals simultaneously receiving medication and/or psychotherapy. Another major purpose of the volume is to identify areas needing research in order to encourage and stimulate individual investigators, as well as funding agencies, in the development of research issues and agendas.

Preparation of this volume has been a labor of love, particularly since the contributors are the leading authorities in the various subareas dealing with the interfaces between exercise and mental health. Most regrettably, during the preparation of the volume one of the contributors, Professor A. H. ("Ish") Ismail, died unexpectedly. We wish to acknowledge Partrick J. O'Connor for revising and editing Professor Ismail's chapter. Shortly after his death a scholarship fund in honor of Professor Ismail was established at Purdue University. All royalties from this volume will be donated to the A. H. Ismail Scholarship Fund.

Multidisciplinary volumes of this nature require the cooperation and support of many individuals and organizations. Each of the authors are identified by a background statement. We also wish to acknowledge support from the Office of Prevention at the National Institute of Mental Health for convening the state-of-the-art-workshop that enabled the authors to discuss the role of exercise in the development and maintenance of mental health.

The entire manuscript was typed initially by Ms. Sharon Ruch, and revisions of selected portions were prepared by Ms. Vinni Pedersen and Ms. Gloria Scalissi. We wish to express our sincere appreciation to each for their expert secretarial contributions. John S. Raglin of the Sport Psychology Laboratory at the University of Wisconsin coordinated the proofing of the manuscript, and he was assisted in this important work by Joan Tincher and David R. Brown. We are particularly indebted to them for their careful attention to reference citations.

Finally, we affirm that prevention, not treatment, offers the best solution to the pandemic mental health problems that characterize modern society—the present volume focuses on one potential coping strategy, *exercise.*

William P. Morgan
Stephen E. Goldston

I

BACKGROUND

1

INTRODUCTION

William P. Morgan and Stephen E. Goldston

The subject of stress has received considerable attention in recent years. It is now widely recognized that prolonged stress may cause a variety of problems such as allergic reactions, dermatitis, gastrointestinal upsets, hypertension, depression, and anxiety. However, we do not know why some individuals seem to be predisposed to respond with such reactions when stressed, nor is it clear why other persons are essentially resistant to the same stressors. Further, it is clear that individual coping strategies can play an important role in the mediation of stress responses.

The Institute of Medicine conducted a project involving the study of research on stress in health and disease in 1981, which resulted in the publication of *Research on Stress and Human Health* (Hamburg, 1981). It is recognized by stress researchers that substantial individual differences exist in the ability to cope with, and tolerate stress, and it is also known that these differences are due in large part to the "coping strategies" employed by stressed individuals. Hamburg (1981) pointed out in the above cited report, however, that ". . . how individuals attempt to cope with stress has been a neglected area of great potential importance." It has also been noted by Hamburg (1981) that a deeper understanding of human coping behavior will be useful in developing both therapeutic and preventive interventions. There is considerable cross-sectional evidence, and some longitudinal data, suggesting that physical activity of a vigorous nature represents a natural, inexpensive, and effective means of coping with mental stress (Morgan, 1981, 1982, 1984, 1985). In a survey of 1,750 primary care physicians, conducted by the *Physician and Sportsmedicine Journal,* (Ryan, 1983) it was found that 85% of the physicians surveyed regularly prescribed exercise in the treatment of depression. While comparable statistics are not available, many psychiatrists, psychologists, and workers in the exercise and sport sciences routinely prescribe exercise for the same reason.

Unfortunately, the actual efficacy of vigorous exercise in the management of anxiety and depression continues to be based largely on indirect and correlational evidence. There have actually been few attempts to demonstrate that exercise intervention, in a controlled, experimental context, results in improved affect. In those cases where experimental trials suggest that exercise is equal or

3

superior to traditional forms of therapy and placebo treatments, there has been no evidence that exercise interventions actually *caused* the observed mood states. In other words, the observed changes have merely been *associated* with the introduction of exercise. While this sort of research has provided important information, the data offer *necessary,* not *sufficient* evidence, in support of the hypothesis that exercise improves mood state.

Little attention has been paid to the question of whether or not an exercise prescription might be contraindicated for some individuals. This is somewhat surprising, given the widespread use of beta-blocking agents in the management of hypertension, and the use of various pharmacologic agents in the treatment of anxiety and depression. Also, little attention has been paid to the issue of exercise "dosage" (i.e., frequency, duration, and intensity).

Furthermore, it is also known that approximately 50% of those individuals who adopt an exercise program discontinue within six to eight weeks. Therefore, even if exercise were proven to possess affective benefits, compliance problems might minimize the overall efficacy of such a coping strategy.

While the *potential role* of exercise as a coping strategy is reasonably well documented, it is necessary that the conditions and circumstances under which such effects occur be delineated in order that exercise intervention effects might be maximized. It is equally important that the limitations and contraindications be elaborated as well. It is known, for example, that an inverse relationship exists between physical fitness and mental health; that is, the higher the physical fitness level, the lower the degree of psychopathology (Morgan, 1981, 1984). Supporting data are largely cross-sectional, but there is limited intervention research supporting the concept of causality. Greist and his associates (1979) at the University of Wisconsin demonstrated, for example, that vigorous aerobic exercise performed for twelve weeks not only reduced depression, but exercise was found to be superior to one form of psychotherapy and equal to a second in its anti-depressant action. This research is significant for several reasons. First, rather than comparing exercise with "nothing" (i.e., a control group), a comparison was made with traditional forms of psychotherapy. Second, considering the time and money required for psychotherapy, in contrast to the "economy" of exercise therapy, an added benefit is seen. Third, all but one of the patients in the running group were free of depressive symptoms at twelve months of follow-up, whereas half of the psychotherapy patients had returned for treatment. This particular investigation, along with subsequent research, is described in this volume.

Physical activity also has potential value because of its efficacy in contrast to drug treatment. The advances in psychopharmacology have played an important role in the treatment of major mental health problems such as depression and anxiety state. Unfortunately, many individuals do not benefit from anti-depressive and/or anti-anxiety medications, and the side-effects and after-effects associated with many psychopharmacologic agents, especially when used with individuals who have mild to moderate disturbances, contraindicate the use of such medications. Reviews of the pharmacology and exercise physiology literatures suggest that attention has not been directed toward an understanding of the interactive or synergistic effects of physical activity and selected psychopharmacologic agents. Another issue concerns the interaction between exercise and various beta-blocking agents. Several years ago it was reported that acute physical activity is comparable to meprobamate, a commonly prescribed tranquilizer at that time, in reducing tension states (deVries and Adams, 1972). This finding has not been replicated, however, and there is also a need to compare exercise with newer benzodiazepine anxiolytics.

The *prevention* of depression and anxiety represents a far more effective health strategy than does *treatment*. This is true whether treatment involves psychotherapy, drug therapy, or a combination of psychotherapy and drugs. Up to this point in time, however, prevention efforts in the mental health field have been limited almost entirely to psychological and social interventions. There is now a research base to permit experimentation with exercise intervention as well, and this volume explores the potential efficacy of exercise.

An extremely perplexing problem, and one that is only partially understood, relates to the matter of exercise compliance. For various reasons, some known and some not known, about fifty percent of all individuals who begin formal exercise programs stop exercising within a short period of time. Indeed, most adherence curves suggest that drop-outs stop exercising before the major psychological and physiological effects can occur (Dishman, 1982; Martin and Dubbert, 1985). This particular problem is examined in Chapters 3 and 5.

NIMH WORKSHOP

The potential and limits of exercise intervention as a means of coping with mental stress were explored in a state-of-the-art workshop which was sponsored by the Office of Prevention of the National Institute of Mental Health and convened in the Spring of 1984 (Morgan, Note 1). This workshop was one of over two dozen such meetings held during the period 1981–1984 to discover the cutting edges of prevention research. The present volume is based on a revised version of the reports given at this gathering. The workshop was based on research evidence, and an effort was made, when and where possible, to consider the potential for application. The workshop was also structured so that resulting materials involving the potential and limits of exercise as a coping strategy could eventually be communicated to primary care physicians, psychologists, psychiatrists, and workers in the field of exercise and sport science, as well as the general public. This volume is based on the workshop papers and discussions.

The workshop was held at the National Institute of Health campus during the period April 25–27, 1984. Papers were prepared and distributed in advance to all participants. A planning and orientation session held on the evening preceeding the opening formal session reinforced the objectives and scope of the workshop, by creating closure and generating a common set of expectancies.

The formal presentation of papers took place over the following day and a half. Since the participants had read each paper in advance, presentors highlighted and summarized the essence of their documents. This format permitted a minimum of 30 minutes focused discussion following each presentation. A more general discussion followed the presentation of each set of papers. Participants joined into working sub-groups during the afternoon of the second day for the purpose of formulating consensus statements regarding "what we know" and "what we need to know" about the relationships between exercise and mental health. The sub-groups dealt with "state-of-the-art" evidence involving anxiety, depression, and programmatic issues. The participants reconvened as a committee of the whole, and spokespersons presented consensus statements for each of the three groups. A verbatim transcript of these statements was prepared and mailed to each participant following the workshop, and he/she was asked to agree or disagree with the statements as formulated. In those instances where disagreement took place, participants indicated the basis for their disagreement, and they also offered suggestions for revision. These consensus statements are presented in Chapter 15, and they reflect the collective and edited versions that eventually emerged.

SUMMARY OF CONTENTS

Following this introductory chapter is an overview of stress, emotions and health by Dr. Charles Spielberger which provides a conceptual basis for the other chapters. Having an agreed upon theoretical foundation is quite important since stress researchers often differ dramatically in their conceptualization and operationalization of these constructs.

Chapter 3 by Dr. Daniel Kirschenbaum deals with the prevention of sedentary lifestyles. Young children are inherently active, but it is widely recognized that progressive inactivity is associated with the aging process. Therefore, rather than focus on the adoption of coping strategies such as regular exercise, a more profitable approach would be to focus our efforts on identification of the factors involved in remaining active.

It is recognized, of course, that many active children go on to become sedentary adults, and the challenge for many workers in the health professions involves the development of an activity plan for individuals in primary or secondary prevention programs. This issue is covered in the following Chapter (4) by Dr. William Haskell. It is imperative that health professionals responsible for developing and supervising exercise programs, adhere to sound guidelines such as those presented in this chapter.

Unfortunately, it is now recognized that adoption of these guidelines will not necessarily prevent all individuals from "dropping out" of exercise programs. For this reason, Chapter 5 by Dr. Rod Dishman deals with the factors involved in exercise adherence. This chapter offers useful insights concerning adherence and drop-out patterns that characterize most adult fitness programs.

This section of the book concludes with Chapter (6) by Dr. Egil Martinsen involving the interaction of exercise and drug therapy in psychiatric patients. This review is relevant since many individuals who are eligible for exercise programs may be receiving various psychopharmacologic agents. While concerns have been raised previously about the wisdom of employing exercise with individuals receiving such medications, this chapter represents the first comprehensive overview on the subject.

The next eight chapters were written by Doctors deVries (7), Morgan (8), Ismail (9), Greist (10), Harris (11), Brown (12), Berger (13), and Sime (14). These contributors possess competencies and research specializations in various fields such as exercise science, psychology, psychiatry, and physical education. The chapters in this section each summarize the results of systematic research programs involving the influence of acute and chronic exercise on anxiety, depression, and personality structure. This section is followed by a Summary Chapter (15) prepared by the editors. The purpose of this chapter is to present a series of consensus statements dealing with the related issues of "what we know" and "what we need to know." The former concerns identify the basis for *intervention efforts,* and the latter provides a *research agenda* for consideration by interested scientists and funding agencies.

The final Chapter (16), prepared by Dr. Michael Sachs, discusses information retrieval models specific to exercise and mental health. This chapter also contains a comprehensive bibliography, including each reference cited in the volume.

II

PRINCIPLES OF EXERCISE INTERVENTION

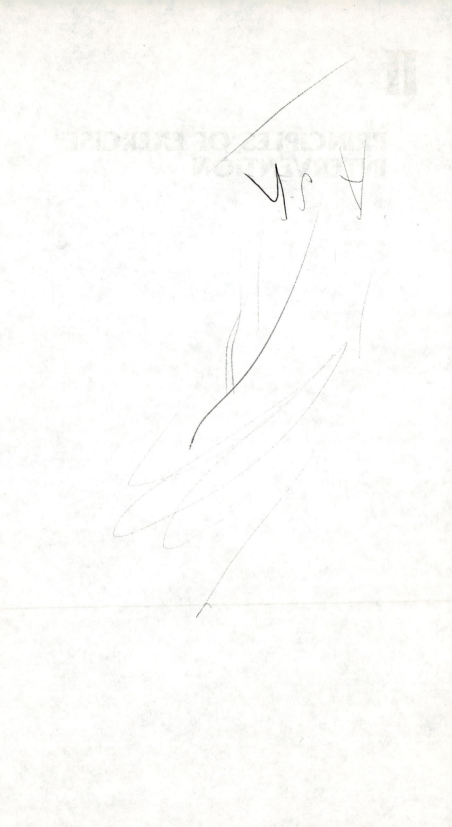

2

STRESS, EMOTIONS AND HEALTH

Charles D. Spielberger

INTRODUCTION

Stress is an integral part of the natural fabric of life and coping with stress is an everyday requirement for normal human growth and development. Even before birth, there is evidence that stress experienced during pregnancy can influence both the mother and the fetus, and may contribute to obstetric complications and birth defects (Edwards & Jones, 1970; Gorsuch & Key, 1974; Spielberger & Jacobs, 1978, 1979). The trauma of birth itself, weaning and toilet training, and the institutionalized demands of society in educating and socializing its young are all unavoidable sources of stress for children and adolescents.

Hurricanes, floods and wars are examples of catastrophic stressors that exert tremendous pressures on large masses of people. Droughts and sudden unseasonal freezes can be especially stressful for farmers, and city dwellers must adjust to street crime, noise and pollution, and crowded living conditions. Taking an examination, speaking in public, pressures and deadlines at work, and stresses associated with marriage, family relationships, retirement, and old age must also be included among the ubiquitous sources of stress. Even holidays and vacations, which are usually regarded as positive events, can be extremely stressful for some people.

The adverse effects of stress on physical health and emotional well-being are increasingly recognized, but there is as yet little agreement among experts on the definition of stress. The prevailing ambiguity and confusion with regard to the nature of stress was noted by the late Professor Hans Selye perhaps the world's foremost medical authority with regard to the effects of stress on bodily processes. In his popular book, *Stress without distress*, Selye gives this definition:

The word "stress", like "success", "failure", or "happiness", means different things to different people so that defining it is extremely difficult. The business man who is under constant pressure from his clients and employees alike, the air traffic controller who knows that a moment of distraction may mean death to hundreds of people, the athlete who wants to win a race, and the husband who helplessly watches as his wife slowly and painfully dies of cancer all suffer from stress. The problems they face are totally different, but medical research has shown that in many respects the body responds in a stereotyped manner, with identical biochemical changes, essentially meant to cope with any type of increased demand upon the human machinery. *(1974, pp. 25-26, emphasis added.)*

From Selye's analysis, it is apparent that stress affects many aspects of life, and that coping with stress is essential for both physical health and effective performance.

The term "stress" is of Latin derivation and was first used in English during the 17th century to describe distress, oppression, hardship and adversity. During the 18th and 19th centuries, popular usage shifted to denote a force, pressure or strong influence acting upon a physical object or person that induced a "strain" in the object. Thus, in common sense terms stress refers to *both* the situations or circumstances that place physical or psychological demand upon an individual and the emotional reactions that are experienced in these situations. The popular usage implies that stress *causes* strain:

Stress → Strain

The concept of stress was introduced into the physical sciences in early investigations of the elastic properties of solid materials in a manner that was generally consistent with popular usage. "Stress" referred to the external pressure or force applied to an object, while "strain" denoted the resulting internal distortion or change in the object. By measuring the force per unit area acting on the object, the relationship between stress and strain can be quantitatively expressed.

Speculation about the effects of life stress on physical and mental illness began in the 19th century. In the early 20th century, a reknowned British physician, Sir William Osler, suggested that stress contributed to the development of heart disease. On the basis of his observations a group of 20 medical doctors suffering from angina pectoris, Osler concluded that these physicians were completely absorbed with "the incessant treadmill of the practice of medicine, and in every one of these men there was an added factor—worry" (1910, pp. 698).

In equating stress with hard work and strain with worry, Osler applied concepts from physics and engineering to problems of human adjustment and behavior. But people are much more complex than inorganic materials; they have the ability to anticipate the future and to interact with and change the environment. Consequently, whether or not a stressful situation produces worry or anxiety will depend on how that situation is perceived or interpreted, and on the individual's coping skills. Thus, some people may react to hard work and responsibility for the health and welfare of others with worry and anxiety, while the same amount and type of work can be challenging and rewarding for others.

Reactions to a situation or event will depend on how the particular circumstances are perceived or appraised. When a person appraises a situation as potentially harmful or threatening, he/she will experience an emotional reaction. Threat appraisals are influenced, of course, by the characteristics of a situation, and objectively dangerous circumstances are generally perceived as threatening by most people. But the thoughts and memories that are stimulated by a particular situation, and an individual's coping skills and previous experience with similar circumstances, can have an even greater impact.

The concept of *threat* is central to Richard Lazarus' (1966) definition of stress as a special kind of transaction between a person and his or her environment. Lazarus defines stress as a complex psychobiological process that consists of three major elements—stressor, threat and emotional reactions. The stress process is initiated by a situation or stimulus that is potentially harmful or dangerous (stressor). If a stressor is interpreted as threatening, an emotional reaction will be evoked. Thus, the stress process involves the following temporal sequence of events:

Stressor → Perception of Threat → Emotional Reaction

The term *stressor* refers to any stimulus situation or event that is objectively characterized by some degree of physical or psychological danger. *Threat* refers to an individual's perception or appraisal of particular circumstances as potentially dangerous or harmful. Whenever an event or situation is seen as threatening, irrespective of whether the danger is real or imagined, the sense of threat will lead to an unpleasant *emotional reaction.*

Emotional reactions may vary in intensity and fluctuate over time as a function of both external stressors, and how they are perceived and appraised. Anxiety and anger are the primary emotional reactions to appraisals of threat and frustration. Anxiety states consist of feelings of tension, apprehension, nervousness and worry, and heightened activation or arousal of the autonomic nervous system. States of anger may vary from feelings of mild irritation and annoyance, to fury and rage, with the level of autonomic arousal corresponding with the intensity of a person's angry feelings.

Everyone feels anxious or angry from time-to-time, but there are substantial differences among people in the frequency and the intensity that such emotions are experienced. The terms *trait anxiety* and *trait anger* refer to individual differences in the proneness to experience these emotions (Spielberger, 1972, 1979). To clarify the distinction between emotional states and personality traits, consider the statement "Mr. Smith is angry". This statement may be interpreted as meaning either that Smith is angry now, at this moment, or that Smith is a chronically angry, hostile person. If Smith is "angry now", this implies that he is presently experiencing some degree of irritation, annoyance or rage.

But if Smith is an "angry person", this indicates that he experiences anger more often than others, that is, Smith has a fiery temper and a low threshold for becoming annoyed and expressing anger.

Over the past two decades, there have been numerous investigations of state and trait anxiety (Spielberger, 1966), but surprisingly little research on anger (Spielberger, Jacobs, Russell, & Crane, 1983). To illustrate the complex relationship between stressors, emotional states, personality traits and adjustments, a conceptual framework based on previous research on anxiety is presented in Figure 1 (Spielberger, 1972, 1979). Each box in the diagram represents a critical element in a stress transaction that links stressors with internal processes and behavioral reactions. The arrows in the diagram refer to the sequence of interactions among the components and to possible influences of one element on another.

The arousal of an anxiety state (A-State), as can be seen in Figure 1, may be initiated by either external or internal stimuli. Any stimulus that is appraised as threatening will evoke an A-State reaction. The intensity and duration of this emotional reaction will be proportional to the amount of threat the situation poses for the individual and the persistence of the evoking stimuli. The objective characteristics of a situation, the thoughts and memories that are elicited or recalled, and the individual's coping skills and previous experience in dealing with similar circumstances all contribute to the appraisal of a situation as more or less threatening.

Individual differences in trait anxiety (A-Trait) also contribute to threat appraisals. While situations that involve physical dangers are interpreted as threatening by most people, circumstances in which personal adequacy is evaluated are more likely to be perceived as threatening by people who are high in A-Trait than by low A-Trait persons. In general, people who are high in trait anxiety are more vulnerable to being evaluated by others because they tend to be low in self-esteem and lack confidence in themselves.

High levels of state anxiety are experienced as extremely unpleasant and motivate behavior designed to eliminate or reduce the anxiety. Two obvious ways of reducing the anxiety aroused by an external danger are simply to avoid the source of danger or to modify the environment so the danger is reduced or eliminated. But people also adjust to stressful situations by engaging in unconscious psychological maneuvers or defenses that alter the way they see a situation without altering the situation itself. Psychological defense mechanisms modify, distort, or render unconscious the feelings, thoughts and memories that would otherwise provoke anxiety. To the extent that a defense mechanism is successful, the stressor will be appraised as less threatening, and there will be a corresponding reduction in A-State intensity.

Research on anger has demonstrated the importance of distinguishing between angry feelings and individual differences in anger proneness as a personality trait (Spielberger et al., 1983). It has also been shown that the expression of anger must be distinguished conceptually and empirically from the experi-

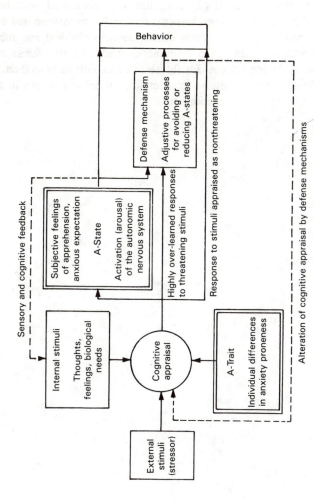

FIGURE 1 A conceptual model of stress and anxiety as a complex psychobiological process. The model posits two anxiety constructs, state anxiety (A-State) and trait anxiety (A-Trait), and specified the relationships between these constructs and external and internal stressors, cognitive appraisal of threat, and coping and defense mechanisms. From Spielberger (1966).

ence of anger as an emotional state, and that expressing anger and holding anger in (suppression) are independent (uncorrelated) psychological dimensions. Evidence of a strong association between anger-hostility and coronary heart disease, and between suppressed anger and elevated blood pressure have also been reported in recent studies (Spielberger, Johnson, Russell, Crane, Jacobs, & Worden, 1984; Spielberger & London, 1982).

Stress, anger and anxiety are widely recognized as contributing to such diverse health problems as insomnia, headaches, skin rashes and even serious medical disorders such as coronary heart disease and cancer. There is also substantial evidence that improved physical fitness is associated with better mental and physical health. Therefore, it seems reasonable to assume that exercise interventions can make an important contribution to physical and mental health, especially, when carried out in combination with effective stress management programs. An important goal for future research will be to evaluate the potential and the limitations of exercise interventions in helping people to cope more effectively with emotional reactions to stress.

3

TOWARD THE PREVENTION OF SEDENTARY LIFESTYLES

Daniel S. Kirschenbaum

Imagine that you are out for a picnic on a pleasant spring day with a group of friends. You have just set out a checkered tablecloth with all manner of your favorite foods. You have situated yourself by the bank of a river, and as you are about to bite into a sandwich a cry is heard from the river. "Help, help!" the screamer yells. Putting down your sandwich, you tear off your shoes and clothes and dive in to rescue a drowning victim, apply artificial respiration, and prepare to return to your picnic. Suddenly two people call out "help, help!" You dive in again and pull them out one on each arm. But as you return there are three or four others calling for help. Again you return, but this time, tired and overwhelmed by several people at once, you let a few slip away. Again, now in larger numbers, people call for help, but you cannot handle very many. You are only one person and you don't even swim very well yourself. Your friends don't swim at all, but as they watch you one has a bright idea. "Why not go upstream and find out who is pushing these people in?" (recounted by Rappaport, 1977, p. 632-origin unknown)

INTRODUCTION

The logic of prevention is well-illustrated by this story of a somewhat strange spring picnic. But, just what is the true benefit of the proverbial "ounce of prevention?" Indeed, that ounce seems very costly to those who dole out the few dollars available for research on health care. Can expenditures on before-the-fact preventive interventions be justified in the present age of retrenchment in federal support (aside from military, that is)? Even more to the point of the present paper, can we justify expenditures to learn how to help people develop more active lifestyles—especially since so many commercial enterprises (e.g., running shoe companies; jogging clothes manufacturers) *seem* to be doing just that and prospering?

17

The purpose of the first section of this paper is to address the question of the value of preventive efforts. Several examples from the medical arena are presented to document the surprisingly potent effects of prevention. The second section considers the rationale for directing preventive interventions at "sedentarianism"—the sedentary lifestyle currently practiced by many millions of Americans. Having made what is hoped to be a convincing argument in support of anti-sedentarianism (the prevention of sedentary lifestyles), the next section presents conceptualizations of prevention. Finally, specific recommendations are reviewed in the fourth section that could facilitate the development of more effective research and intervention on anti-sedentarianism.

WHY WE NEED PREVENTION

Cleanliness Is Next to Healthiness

Many decades before medical authorities accepted germ theory in the early 19th century, health oriented officials took steps to eradicate *miasmas,* or noxious odors associated with sewage (Bloom, 1984). Even without the benefit of knowing that germs cause disease, the teachings of Hippocrates and others led to widespread acceptance of the belief that specific miasmas like the "bad air" (malaria) associated with swamps and sewage were responsible for most infectious diseases. These beliefs led to efforts to improve sanitation which, in turn, greatly reduced thyphoid fever, yellow fever, tuberculosis, cholera, and infant and maternal mortality. For example, by 1800 maternal mortality had been lowered to one-seventh of its 1750 level.

Of course, the improvements in sanitary conditions often occurred mainly in the living conditions of the wealthier classes in the last 200 hundred years. For example, consider the following graphic description of the unbelievable conditions in which many thousands of immigrants found themselves as they contributed to the industrial revolution in the middle and late 1800's in England: "The infrequency of sewage and garbage removal, as well as the neglected state of the courts and alleys around which the houses were built, gave rise to the practice of using them as places of deposit for all the residents of a given court. As a result, there was scarcely a court that was not occupied by a communal cesspool or dunghill. Houses in the poorer districts had no water closets, and many had no privies. These conditions were not restricted to the homes of the working classes, but they were worst there. In "Little Ireland" in Manchester, there were two privies to 250 people. Nearby Ashton had one district with only two privies for 50 families, and such instances could easily be repeated for other communities. Instead of water closets or privies, there was a "necessary," a kind of tub that had to be emptied every morning. Even with this facility, the situation was grim. In one Manchester district the needs of some 7000 people were supplied by 33 "necessaries," that is, supplied after a fashion. Since there was in most cases no access to the back yard except through the house, all the dirt and filth had to be carried through rooms, passageways, doorways, and over pavements, which were defiled as a result. This cloacal inferno was even intensified by the rapid migration during the 1840's of thousands of starving Irish who streamed through the port of Liverpool to huddle in the cellars and hovels of factory towns and cities like Birmingham, Bristol, Leets, Manchester, and others.

The overcrowding in these dwellings can be imagined. Manchester had 1500 cellars where three persons, 738 where four, and 281 where five slept in one bed. In Bristol there were 2800 families, of whom 46 percent had one room each. Liverpool had 40,000 people who lived in cellars and 60,000 in close courts as described. These figures must be seen against the background information that out of a population of 223,054 in the 1841 census, 160,000 belonged to the working classes. In short, more than 70 percent were workers and more than 60 percent of these lived in crowded, dirty, unsanitary conditions (Rosen, 1958, pp. 205–206).''

Vaccinations and Further Improvements in Sanitation in the 20th Century

In this century, many steps have been taken to improve sanitation across socioeconomic stratas, to isolate disease carriers when treatments have been ineffective or long in duration, and to develop preventive medical vaccinations. Small pox, diptheria, diarrheal diseases of infancy, tuberculosis, influenza, measles, and polimyelitis have become either completely eliminated, nearly so, or much better controlled as a result of these efforts. For example, the *1979 Surgeon General's Report on Health Promotion and Disease Prevention* clearly shows that the preventive medical efforts implemented during this century have paid off in the savings of literally millions of lives (Califano, 1979).

It is important to emphasize that these improvements resulted from improvements in hygiene, diet, and preventive medical care. These dramatic changes were *not* due to advances in biomedical knowledge regarding the treatment of infectious diseases (Leventhal, Zimmerman, & Gutmann, 1984; Thomas, 1977). Furthermore, we should certainly begin recognizing that the two identified major causes of death in the last year (and to date) are unlikely to be "cured" by advances in biomedical research—at least in the forseeable future. For people who develop most forms of cancer and heart disease, medical science can offer only technologies which decelerate disease progression (to minimal extents in many cases) or allow people to maintain a reasonable quality of life while moving inexorably toward early death (Thomas, 1977). Paradoxically, the vast majority of dollars spent on health concerns goes to medical care for the sick. In 1973, for example, 92-93% of the $83 billion spent for health care in the United States was spent on medical treatment for the sick; 4-5% for biomedical research; 2% on public health sanitation measures (e.g., rodent control); and less than one half of 1% on health education (Marshall, 1977).

Prevention by Legislation

The Case of Motorcycle Helmets   Seven times as many people who are in motorcycle accidents get injured compared to the percentage of injuries resulting from automobile accidents (Watson, Zador, & Wilks, 1980, 1981). This resulted in more than 4000 deaths and 350,000 injuries sustained in motorcycle accidents in 1977 alone (Bloom, 1984). In the mid-1970's virtually all states enacted laws requiring motorcycle riders to wear helmets. Approximately 30% fewer people died from motorcycle accidents in the year immediately after these laws were passed. However, lobbying by the American Motorcyclist Association and changes in federal mandates resulted in the repeal of these laws in 26 states between 1976 and 1978. An increase in motorcycle fatalities and injuries rose by a substantial amount in 23 of the 26 states that had repealed the law. Watson and associates (1980) showed that there was a 38% increase in fatalities in those states that repealed the law compared to geographically and demographically similar states that retained the law. All of this makes a great deal of sense given the evidence that mortality rates are twice as high in unhelmeted compared to helmeted accident victims.

The Case of Safety Belt Usage   More than 50% of the children born in 1972 will sustain injuries at sometime in their lives as a result of an automobile accident (Kahn, 1973). Fortunately, wearing a seat belt could reduce traffic fatalities by 25% and traffic injuries by 50% (Geller, Johnson, & Pelton, 1982). Unfortunately, observations obtained by the U.S. Department of Transportation of more than 150,000 drivers in 19 metropolitan areas from November 1977 through November 1979 showed that "safety belt usage by drivers is down from 14% in 1978 to 10.9% in 1979 (Geller, Paterson, & Talbot, 1982). Several major studies have now shown that various forms of prompts and contingencies can dramatically improve this low percentage of safety belt usage (see Geller, 1983).

Most of the larger industrialized countries have used this information and established seat belt laws to prevent many of the adverse effects of traffic accidents. For example, if vehicle occupants are observed by police to be not wearing seat belts, then they are fined in Canada, England, France, Germany, and Sweden. Several major American industries have developed incentive programs to increase seat belt usage because of the substantial savings in insurance costs resulting from such programs (Geller, 1983; Gellar et al., 1982). At a federal level, however, our country has opted for less preventive health and more industrial profit in the most recent past. The Carter administration mandated equipping all new 1983 U.S. vehicles with passive restraints (automatic seat belts or air bags). To the delight of the automotive industry, the Reagan administration rescinded that legislation.

The above examples clearly document the efficiency and effectiveness of a variety of preventive efforts. Many other examples exist (see Bloom, 1984), but these make the necessary point quite clearly: It is very apparent that large-scale preventive interventions can be well worth the expenditures they require in terms of time and effort. What is needed to begin such efforts, in addition to an adequate level of funding and person-power, is a clear rationale for focusing preventive efforts on a particular behavior, problem, or aspect of living. The rationale must show a clear relationship between the proposed focal aspect of living and health outcomes. Sanitary environmental conditions, vaccinations for various diseases, use of motorcycle helments, and use of seatbelts had all dem-onstrated their efficacy as preventive strategies before community—and society-wide preventive programs were launched focused on them. Let us now consider whether a similar empirical justification currently exists for the advocacy of anti-sedentarianism.

A RATIONALE FOR ANTI–SEDENTARIANISM

They are fatally mistaken who think that while they strive with their minds that they may suffer their bodies to stagnate in luxury and sloth. Henry David Thoreau (1840, p. 42)

The wisdom of Thoreau is not an adequate reason to advocate the radical alteration of lifestyles as a means of preventing various health problems. Fortu-nately, the data have been accumulating rapidly which provide more objective support for Thoreau's assertion.

Martin and Dubbert (1982) summarized much of the current evidence on the effects on physical well-being of the practice of systematic, regular aerobic exercises (15+ minutes per session, 3+ sessions per week, in which repetitive isorhythmic activities are focal). They reported that such exercise programs have improved cardiovascular efficiency and modified cardiovascular risk pro-files in healthy people, as well as in individuals at high risk for cardiovascular disease, coronary patients, and borderline hypertensives. Getting coronary pa-tients to engage in regular and sustained exercise programs has also been linked with improvements in recovery, such as shorter hospitalization and decreased perceived exertion. All of these findings are extremely important in view of the increasing proportion of deaths in this country that are attributable to cardiovas-cular disease.

Focusing treatment for obesity on increasing energy expenditure, in addi-tion to decreasing energy intake, also appears to yield important payoffs (Mar-tin & Dubbert, 1982). Treatment outcome studies with children (Epstein, Wing, Koeske, Ossip, & Beck, 1982) and adults (Dahlkoetter, Callahan & Linton, 1979; Stalonas, Johnson, & Christ, 1978) indicates that the addition of exercise programs is an active contributor to the efficacy of treatment. Martin and Dub-bert (1982) aptly noted that these effects may be due to reduced appetite, adap-tive modification of physiological adjustment to dieting, use of exercise as a coping strategy or timeout mechanism, and the potentially stress reducing ef-fects of exercising. Regardless of the mechanism, considering the highly refractory nature of obesity and its substantial health risks, the beneficial effects associated with exercise represents one of the most clinically significant findings for the treatment of obesity that has been accumulated in the past two decades.

A great many additional benefits have been suggested and associated with lifestyles that include regular programs of physical exercise (see reviews by Folkins & Sime, 1981; Morgan, 1984, 1985; Weinstein & Meyers, 1983). Increasing physical activity *may:* prolong life among diabetics, improve intellectual functioning among elderly people, improve work performance, ameliorate sleep disorders, enhance sexual enjoyment, decrease depression and anxiety, and improve self-concept. Increasingly sophisticated studies are emerging which are beginning to suggest that many of these possibilities are probabilities. For example, Doyne, Chambless, and Beutler (1983) recently demonstrated that clients with major depressive disorder could improve their affective states substantially following the introduction of an aerobic training program. This finding is noteworthy not because of its originality (see Morgan, 1984), but because it demonstrated effects due to exercising while controlling for client expectancies and amount of contact with therapists.

In addition to establishing the real and probable benefits of exercising, part of the rationale for the prevention of sedentarianism must include documentation of the pervasiveness of the problem in this regard. In other words, we must consider the extent to which people currently practice sedentary lifestyles. In a recent paper, John Martin appropriately characterized and summarized the current lifestyle practices in America:

> *Studies have shown that virtually everyone believes that exercise, like democracy, is a good thing. Regrettably, the majority of individuals become merely approving spectators to each . . . As poor as our voting participation is (65% of eligible Americans actually vote), our regular exercise participation in the U.S. (37%) is worse! (1981, p. 3)*

Not only do 63% of Americans fail to exercise regularly, a series of 1978 Harris polls (cited by Martin & Dubbert, 1982) indicate that 45% may not exercise at all. Furthermore, approximately one-half of the people who begin health-related exercise programs re-join the ranks of their more sedentary peers within 6 months of beginning such efforts (Dishman, 1984). This difficulty in "treating" sedentarianism suggests that preventive efforts may prove more cost-efficient than remedial efforts and that further developments in research and conceptualizations may be needed to advance both remedial and preventive approaches.

The final section of this paper will attempt to refine current views of the nature of the problem of sedentarianism, leading to practical suggestions for improving the efficacy of preventive programs targeted to anti-sedentarianism.

Before providing those suggestions, however, it is necessary to review the options available for preventive interventions. For now, it seems safe to conclude that : (a) prevention is a practical and very useful approach to reducing various health problems, and (b) sedentarianism is a health concern of sufficient impact to justify considering approaches to prevention that could reduce its prevalence in this country.

CONCEPTS AND APPROACHES IN PREVENTION

Three Types

There are many dozens of ways of operationalizing the basic concept of prevention. Gerald Caplan's book, *Principles of Preventive Psychiatry* (1964) brought the concept of preventive intervention into the modern mental health movement by defining the three major types of prevention.

He defined *tertiary prevention* as the reduction of problems in an entire community (i.e., large scale amelioration) by intervening with people who have already developed serious problems in living. This idea is closest to traditional health care delivery, so much so that Bloom (1984) suggested that it is equivalent to rehabilitation. However, one difference is that the term tertiary prevention directs attention to the impact on the community of such rehabilitative efforts. An approach to anti-sedentarianism that is an example of tertiary prevention is an exercise class provided for all coronary patients in a particular hospital who had practiced a sedentary lifestyle prior to their heart attacks. This large scale rehabilitation effort might decrease the incidence of sedentarianism among the patients in the hospital and others in the community who observed the effects they achieved.

Secondary prevention refers to reducing the rate of problems in a community by intervening at the early stages of the development of problems in living. This could include, for example, providing young executives in a business with easy access to health club facilities, time off from work for working out, and otherwise encouraging those at high risk for life-long sedentarianism (e.g., young people who have already developed relatively sedentary lifestyles) to develop regular exercise habits. Finally, *primary prevention* is the lowering of the rate of problems in a community "by counteracting harmful circumstances before they have a chance to produce illness" (Caplan,1964, p. 26). Thus, the major difference between primary and secondary prevention is that the former acts before-the-fact, or before-the-emergence of the problem, while secondary prevention amounts to early intervention, usually with young people, after the problem has already emerged in an early stage. Primary prevention, therefore, can be, and often is, directed at "high risk" groups, as reflected in the following carefully considered definition of primary prevention applied to mental health:

Primary prevention encompasses those activities directed to specifically identified vulnerable high-risk groups within the community who have not been labeled as psychiatrically ill and for whom measures can be undertaken to avoid the onset of emotional disturbance and/or to enhance their level of positive mental health. (Goldston, 1977, p. 27)

Focus, Timeframe, and Target Population

The specific incarnation of a prevention program depends in large part on the central focus or goal of the intervention, the timeframe utilized, and dimension of the target population (Cowen, 1980; Jason & Glenwick, 1980). Table 1 presents a 4 × 2 × 5 (focus × timeframe × dimension of target population) matrix of the variations in primary and secondary prevention programming that could be utilized in efforts to encourage anti-sedentarianism.

Focus: The focus dimension was distilled from a variety of papers on the extant practices and future possibilities for primary prevention (e.g., Cowen, 1977, 1980; Jason & Glenwick, 1980; Goldston, 1977). Many programs have focused on methods of presenting information to individuals, groups, and larger segments of the population. These are sometimes referred to as educational programs or mass media campaigns. The users of this focus hope that the information will help people modify their behaviors or change their laws or environments to prevent specific problems from developing or worsening. Billboards and commercials warning us about the dangers of cigarette smoking, driving while drunk, and stress are common examples of this dimension of focus.

Prevention programs can also attempt to improve skills or competencies, such as social problem solving skills or self-control skills. Programs have at-

TABLE 1   Key dimensions in primary and secondary prevention

	Focus							
	Provide information		Improve competencies		Improve adjustment to stressors		Modify environments	
Audience	Acute	Chronic	Acute	Chronic	Acute	Chronic	Acute	Chronic
Individual								
Group								
Organization								
Community								
Society								

tempted to train elementary school children in these skills, including several large scale efforts directed at unselected groups of children (e.g., Weissberg et al., 1981) and secondary prevention programs aimed at children with mild to moderate behavioral-emotional difficulties (e.g., Kirschenbaum, Pedro-Carroll, & DeVoge, 1983). In a related vein, programs have focused on helping people learn how to cope with impending or existing crises or stressors. These programs use known or specifically anticipated stressful events as the major impetus for the intervention. Thus, programs aimed at preparing children for hospitalization and surgery (e.g., Peterson & Shigetomi, 1981; Zastowny, Kirschenbaum, & Meng, in press) and dental treatment (e.g., Klorman et al., 1980) are not primarily directed at generalized skill building. Rather, they are aimed at reducing the potentially adverse impact of stressors.

Finally, preventive interventions can focus on modifying environments. Efforts could be directed to change the size of elementary school classrooms or the use of certain rules and organizational structures to reduce the frequency of classroom disruptions, enhance self-control, and improve affect (Humphrey, 1984). An example from a different domain of behavior concerns a significant ecological problem—littering. Geller, Mann, & Brasted (1977) rotated ordinary and artistically designed litter drums every 5–8 weeks for a year. The creative containers were shaped like birds, brightly painted, and contained a litter-reduction message. The colorful containers attracted much more litter than the ordinary drums (15 versus 9 pounds per week)—thereby effectively preventing a good deal of littering (approximately 312 pounds per year, per container).

Timeframe: Preventive interventions can vary in duration, in addition to focus. Bloom (1984) described the *milestone* approach to prevention as providing services to people "when they reach a particular, predefined point—or when they undergo some particular stressful life event (p. 200)." Examples of the milestone approach, which are always delivered in an acute, time-limited fashion, include preparatory programs for surgical and dental procedures (e.g., Kendall et al., 1978; Klorman et al., 1980; Melamed & Siegel, 1975; Zastowny et al., in press). These programs can focus on improving adjustment to stressors, but they can also focus on providing information only, improving general competencies, and modifying environments. For example, most extant programs designed to prevent maladjustment among children undergoing hospitalization for surgery focus on providing information (Peterson & Ridley-Johnson, 1980).

Quite a few preventive interventions use a much more extended, or chronic, timeframe. Many early secondary prevention programs for children, for example, attempt to build competencies and improve adjustment via therapy and consultation delivered over one, and often several, years (e.g., Cowen et al., 1975; Kirschenbaum et al., 1983). Programs targeted to improve the ecology and safety (e.g., litter reduction; recycling; seat belt usage) often include long-term interventions and evaluation (as in the attractive litter container example mentioned earlier, Geller et al., 1977). The programs of longer duration often attempt to change more chronic or refractory conditions and they tend to be more likely to evaluate such efforts for generalized effects (e.g., Geller, 1983).

Target Population: Jason and Glenwick (1980) made it clear that prevention programs can be targeted to individuals, groups, organizations, communities, or societies. Many programs, especially competency building or adjustment programs, train individuals. However, a number of preventive efforts have targeted naturally interacting groups, such as classrooms and families. Kirschenbaum, Harris, and Tomarken (1984), for example, showed that including overweight parents in weight control groups with their overweight children decreased attrition and facilitated a cooperative pattern of family weight control, compared to having overweight children and their overweight parents work more independently.

Larger groups, or organizations, can also benefit from preventive interventions. Entire schools, companies, community mental health centers, residence halls, and hospitals have received interventions designed to improve attendance, job performance, and reduce the probability of a variety of disruptions (Jason & Glenwick, 1980). Many of these efforts focus on modifying environments. For example, Jason & Glenwick (1980, p. 21) reviewed the results of two studies that modified nursing home environments. In efforts designed to prevent social isolation and concomitant mental/physical deterioration, researchers placed puzzles, other equipment, and refreshments into lounge areas. These environmental changes effectively and sharply increased social interaction by the nursing home residents.

Even larger scale efforts have been aimed at entire communities or societies. These often involve mass media educational efforts designed to promote attitudinal or behavioral changes, such as decreasing smoking, decreasing littering, decreasing drunk driving, and increasing social support via volunteer work. Some examples of these programs will be presented in the final section of this paper when specific approaches to anti-sedentarianism are considered.

Guiding Strategy for Implementation

The foregoing analysis showed that some preventive programs can be described within a 4 × 2 × 5 matrix (focus × timeframe × target population). Additional dimensions could be incorporated (see Cowen, 1980), but the 40 cells described in the present model provide a good sampling of the major options available to those interested in the primary and secondary prevention of sedentarianism.

Each preventive program, regardless of its specific focus, timeframe, or target population, evolves within 4-stages of a general strategy:

Stage 1. Identify a problem of sufficient importance to justify the development of a preventive intervention program.

Stage 2. Develop reliable methods for diagnosing the presence/absence/degree of the problem so that target populations and the efficacy of interventions can be assessed accurately.

Stage 3: Using epidemiological, correlation, quasi-experimental, and experimental methodology, identify likely pathways of the origin and development of the problem.

Stage 4: Mount, evaluate, and then refine and further develop experimental preventive intervention programs based on the results of Stages 2 and 3. (adapted from Bloom, 1984, p. 198).

Many efforts designed to prevent problems of all sorts have omitted one of more of these stages. Many expensive educational campaigns fill commercial television airways with obstensibly little regard for their actual effects on specific target populations. Thus, television commercials direct us to think of behavioral-emotional problems as analogous to medical problems. This propagation of the medical model of psychological problems has persisted for two decades, heedless of findings indicating the adverse effects of such conceptualizations (e.g., Farina, Fisher, Getter, & Fischer, 1978) and campaigns (Sarbin & Mancuso, 1970; Morrison, 1980). The next section of this paper is devoted to an analysis of existing conceptualizations and interventions targeted at anti-sedentarianism. It is offered to help avoid some of the mistakes made by campaigns for prevention launched in other areas and to help improve the efficacy of existing work on anti-sedentarianism.

TOWARD EFFECTIVE PROGRAMS
FOR ANTI–SEDENTARIANISM

It is important to consider the current status of anti-sedentarianism from the perspective of the major questions raised in each of the 4-stages of the general strategy for prevention. This analysis will allow for consideration of which of the 40 types (cells) of preventive programs are being used currently and which should be developed or improved.

Stage 1. *Is sedentarianism an important enough problem to justify the development of preventive intervention programs?* The previous section on the rationale for anti-sedentarianism clearly implicated sedentary lifestyles in the development of cardiovascular problems and obesity. The section also showed that lifestyles incorporating vigorous and regular exercising probably can help prevent these and other problems (e.g., behavioral-emotional troubles), while potentially promoting a higher quality of life. Certainly these are important goals. The first section of this paper further justifies work on anti-sedentarianism by demonstrating the cost-effectiveness of prevention programming.

Stage 2. *Can we reliably and accurately assess sedentarianism?* A recent paper by Thompson & Martin (1984) clearly documented that a number of effective and efficient procedures, several with existing norms, can be used to assess cardiovascular fitness. There are also some questionnaires that have established track records for assessing relevant cognitive aspects of sedentarianism, most notably the "Self-motivation Questionnaire" developed by Dishman and his colleagues (Dishman & Ickes, 1981; Dishman, Ickes, & Morgan, 1980). However, these procedures can assess only some aspects of sedentarianism, and they do that only indirectly. Measures of physical fitness, for example, provide indices of fitness relative to normative groups. They do not show how frequently a person exercises vigorously or uses stairs instead of elevators. Even baseline to post-treatment assessments of fitness provide only one correlate of the cognitive-behavioral-physical activity changes that are generally targeted in anti-sedentarianism programs (e.g., Keir & Lanzon, 1980; Heyer, Nash, McAlister, Maccoby, & Farquhar, 1980).

Stage 3. *Do we know the likely pathways of the origins and development of sedentarianism?* We know surprisingly little about this crucial phase of prevention applied to sedentary lifestyles. There have been some relevant, but largely correlational, studies that describe, primarily, who is likely to discontinue vigorous exercise programs, i.e., the development and maintenance of anti-sedentarianism among high risk adults. Since much of this work has been conducted by Dishman, and since this work is described in Chapter V, the present summary will be brief (see, also, Dishman, 1984; Martin & Dubbert, 1982).

It seems that among the 50% of the population who are likely to quit their exercise programs within the first six months there are a disproportionate number of people at "high risk" for significant cardiovascular problems (e.g., people who are overweight, smoke, and less knowledgeable about health risks). Furthermore, various social-environmental and cognitive-behavioral factors contribute substantially to likelihood of recidivism in such efforts (e.g., lack of social support; selecting unenjoyable, solitary, and inconvenient exercise programs; choosing only difficult and inflexible exercise goals and plans).

This work has led to a valuable realization that should be applied to conceptualizations of secondary prevention programs designed to change the exercise habits of high risk adults:

> *Exercise can, perhaps, be likened in many respects to attempts at dieting, quitting smoking, reducing alcohol intake or other "New Years Resolutions" by which people attempt to consciously change what has for them become a behavioral habit unconducive to their health or well-being! People start, but they don't finish (pp. 2–3). Rod K. Dishman (1984)*

Stage 4. *Do we know how to mount and evaluate experimental anti-sedentarianism programs based on extant knowledge of this problem?* There are two answers to this bottom-line question. First, there are sufficient measures of physical fitness, as well as measures of related cognitive-behavioral variables (e.g., self-motivation; depression), to assess some key outcomes for which anti-sedentarianism programs are directed. However, the above material regarding Stage 2 make it clear that further work in this area is sorely needed. Second, regarding intervention, we know more about what *not* to do than about what to do at this juncture. The major realization derived from Stage 3 indicates that interventions which focus primarily on "providing information" should prove quite ineffectual in altering sedentarianism among high risk adults. In fact, "previous research has indicated that well-conducted mass media campaigns directed at large, open populations can effectively transmit information, alter some attitudes, and produce small shifts in behavior, such as effecting choices among consumer products, but has failed to demonstrate that media alone can substantially influence more complex behavior" (Meyer, Nash, McAlister, Maccoby, & Farquhar, 1980, p. 130). This conclusion does not mean that intensive public campaigns cannot produce benefits to some of the people some of the time. The evidence suggests that more intensive, group—rather than only community targeted, health promotion campaigns can produce significant, usually small, improvements in various health risk factors (e.g., Meyer *et al.*, 1980). Perhaps people who are currently non-sedentary (e.g., children; non-obese casual exercisers) can be influenced to intensify their efforts via individual, group, or even community-society level campaigns. The question remains, nonetheless, how should secondary prevention programs for anti-sedentarianism be implemented? Furthermore, what are some promising strategies for primary prevention?

RECOMMENDATIONS TOWARD EFFECTIVE ANTI–SEDENTARIANISM

Primary Prevention

The very formidable costs and unproven effects of primary prevention for anti-sedentarianism make secondary prevention efforts more easily justified. Also, risk profiles for cardiovascular disorders and depression help more firmly establish that people who are currently rather sedentary and depressive (or anxious) are especially vulnerable to very adverse effects associated with long-term sedentarianism. Thus, most attempts at anti-sedentarianism in the near future probably should focus on secondary prevention, using groups at high risk for sustained sedentarianism and likely to be adversely affected by same.

This recommendation does not imply that primary prevention programming should cease entirely. It is very probable that some relatively inexpensive strategies could significantly deter at least some individuals from sedentarianism. Unfortunately, little extant empirical evidence is available to direct these efforts. It seems likely, for example, that certain media campaigns (i.e., focusing on providing information) may prove effective for certain sub-populations, such as children or mildly-to-moderately active young adults. It would be very useful, therefore, to conduct analyses of the specific effects of various types of programs that provide information on sedentarianism to these sub-populations. This point advocates refined program by person analyses. It also calls for evaluations of preventive programming on those heretofore neglected sub-populations, in addition to continuing studies on high risk groups that are quite difficult to change (Meyer et al., 1980).

One focus for primary prevention programming has already demonstrated its promise as an efficient and surprisingly effective approach at least for inducing some changes in sedentarianism. Several clinical trials and at least one experiment have used environmental modifications targeted to communities (Brownell et al., 1980) and societies (e.g., Kier & Lauzon, 1980). For example, Brownell et al., (1980) placed a large sign ($3' \times 3^{1/2}'$) at several choice points in which pedestrians could take either stairs or escalators to reach their destinations. In their first of two studies, the sign more than doubled (i.e., significantly increased) use of stairs by obese and nonobese white men and women who were both under and over 30. The use of stairs decreased to near-baseline levels when the sign was withdrawn, but stair usage significantly and immediately increased again on the first day the sign was returned. A replication again showed an immediate substantial impact of the sign that was largely maintained one month after withdrawal, but not at 3 months. Unfortunately, obese people did not respond differentially to the presence or absence of the sign in the replication study.

Perhaps such environmental changes could induce some people to lead more active lives. The previously noted findings on exercise programs for high risk adults (Dishman, 1984) make it unlikely that many high risk people would change substantially as a function of such interventions (e.g., recall the non-significant effects for obese people in the Brownell et al., replication study). However, environmental modifications may be an inexpensive way to facilitate the effectiveness of more intensive individual or group targeted secondary prevention programs emphasizing "lifestyle exercising" (e.g., Epstein et al., 1982). These could produce promising results even for high risk groups. Furthermore, if communities embrace such concepts, that could promote larger scale adoption of inexpensive but effective means to support anti-sedentarianism. This could become operationalized in further environmental modifications. Thus, a more "anti-sedentary future" could include more attractive stairwells, perhaps with built-in sound systems, fewer escalators and elevators, tolls for using escalators and elevators, "park and walk" programs for commuters replacing extant "park and ride" campaigns, and so on.

Secondary Prevention

Most of what has been learned about sedentarianism can be used to develop potentially very effective secondary prevention interventions. The justification for such efforts has been clearly established (re: physical health) and guidelines for target populations and focus on intervention are easily derived from a substantial empirical foundation.

Regarding the latter issues, the most appropriate dimensions for target population are "individual" and "group". The work of Dishman (e.g., 1984) and others (e.g., Meyer et al., 1980) show that promoting anti-sedentarianism to people at risk for early cardiovascular problems mandates new conceptualizations of the problem and the intervention. Instead of viewing anti-sedentarianism for this sub-population as a problem that is readily modified via mass media campaigning, it should be viewed and treated as a highly refractory self-regulatory problem.

Viewing sedentary lifestyles as a self-regulatory problem means that we can apply the substantial literature accumulated on behavioral self-regulation to refining methods of improving and maintaining exercise habits. Exercising is a self-regulated problem because it involves regulating one's goal-directed behaviors without immediate external constraints (Kanfer & Karoly, 1972). Furthermore, for many individuals at high risk for coronary problems (e.g., obese, already somewhat sedentary, adults), improving exercise habits presents a conflict between immediate short-term goals (e.g., staying relaxed and comfortable; time pressures, avoiding the stress of dieting) and long-term goals (e.g., sustained good health). This defines anti-sedentarianism as a "special" type of self-regulatory problem, the tolerance of noxious stimulation variant of self-control.

Table 2 presents the 5 phases of self-regulation and their defining features. It is beyond the scope of this paper to review, in detail, each aspect of self-regulation (see Kirschenbaum, 1984a). However, drawing on the previous work in this area, a set of recommendations for interventions for reducing sedentarianism can be offered pertaining to each phase of self-regulation.

Self-control (and self-regulation, more generally) involves complex interactions between cognitions (e.g., goal-setting; planning; self-evaluation), affect (i.e., emotional states), physiology (e.g., strength), and environmental variables. In a recent paper (Kirschenbaum, 1984a), these complex relationships were described in five sequential phases: (1) problem identification; (2) commitment; (3) execution; (4) environmental management; (5) generalization. This analysis, based on work by Kanfer & Karoly (1972; Karoly, 1977) and others (e.g., Mahoney & Thoresen, 1974), can be applied directly to the problem of anti-sedentarianism. In so doing, it helps suggest appropriate foci, timeframes, and target population dimensions for secondary prevention programming.

Problem Identification

It is probably necessary, but not sufficient, for individuals to realize the long-term impact of sedentarianism and, conversely, the many potential benefits of more active lifestyles, including effects on mood states. This information should be communicated clearly and dramatically, using statistics (e.g., Surgeon General's Report) as well as personalized appeals (e.g., from coronary patients who regret their histories of sedentarianism and individuals who have

TABLE 2 Defining features of 5 phases of self-regulation

Phases	Features	Results
Problem identification	Initial identification of self-regulatory problems.	Change is possible
Commitment	Development of initial goals and performance promises.	Change is desirable
Execution	Starting to change.	Change can be achieved through self-monitoring, self-evaluation, and self-consequation.
Environmental management	Modifying social and physical environment to maximize the probability of goal-attainment.	Change can be facilitated in a supportive environment.
Generalization	Maintaining change over time and across settings.	Change can be maintained by developing an obsessive-compulsive style of self-regulating.

enjoyed several specific emotional as well as physical health benefits of active lifestyles).

Commitment

It is clear that the amount of expressed desire to improve physical fitness can predict perseverance in exercise programs of various sorts (Dishman & Ickes, 1981; Dishman et al., 1980). It may be helpful to incorporate "milestone" or acute timeframes in preventive programs, in part, because of these findings. People may be more likely to commit to a goal when they reach a certain milestone, like their 30th or 40th birthdays or a new, sedentary, job.

Several persuasive tactics can also intensify that commitment. For example, Janis and colleagues (see Janis & Mann, 1977) have had people complete "balance sheets" in which they identify many positive and negative outcomes that might result from achieving specific goals. Table 3 presents an example on a balance sheet completed by someone who was deciding whether or not to increase his jogging from once every week or two to 3 days per week. As shown in Figure 1, this procedure seems to help people increase their commitment and, thereby, improve the likelihood of achieving desired anti-sedentarianism outcomes. Additional findings from literatures on goal-setting and planning can also be incorporated to maximize the probability of success (Kirschenbaum, 1985; Locke et al., 1981).

Execution

With a self-regulatory problem identified and a commitment developed to modify it, the active change process or execution phase begins. This process is frequently conceptualized in cybernetic terms (Carver, 1979; Kanfer & Karoly, 1972). Individuals are presumed, for example, to self-monitor (systematically attend to and record target behaviors) self-evaluate (compare performance to goals), self-consequate (self-reward if goals are achieved; self-punish if goals

TABLE 3   An example of a decision balance sheet: GOAL, "To increase my jogging to 3 days per week (from once every week or two)"

Result	Positive effects	Negative effects
Tangible gains and losses for me	Improved health in the short run	Cost of new shoes and other equipment
	Increased life span	Lots of effort
	Improved energy for work	Less time to relax in other ways
	Improved looks (weight loss)	Pain and potential injuries
	Decreased depression and tension	
	Participate in competitive races	
	More health conscious	
	Able to eat rich foods more often	
Tangible gains and losses involving others	Improved ability at team sports	Less time for family and friends
	Better model for friends and family	More complaining to others about injuries
	Meet other joggers	Less tolerance of others (e.g., smokers)
	Better mood when interacting with others (better listener)	
Self-approval or self-disapproval	Proud of self (improved self-concept)	Get tougher on self in other areas
	Less guilt about eating	Become addicted to running
	Increased confidence for trying other difficult tasks	
Approval by others or disapproval by others	Compliments from family	Concern from others about addition to running
	Compliments from friends	Annoyance from family about decreased time
	Compliments from co-workers	Concern from others about more interest in exercise than work
	Recognition from others (if successful at races)	Annoyance from others due to my super-health consciousness (e.g., "party pooper")
	Envy from other if very successful at races	

are not achieved), and, in so doing, continually strive to modify target behaviors.

Many studies have helped to refine these conceptualizations, thereby clarifying principles of self-regulation. For example, one important principle that has emerged from recent research is: "Differential expectancies and self-monitoring interact with task mastery to affect self-regulation" (Kirschenbaum, 1984a). Studies have shown, for example, that self-monitoring successes, not failures, often improves performance of difficult tasks (e.g., Kirschenbaum & Karoly, 1977). This finding has been applied to sport contexts and the results indicate that when people are novices in sports like golf (Johnston-O'Connor & Kirschenbaum, 1986) and bowling (Kirschenbaum, Ordman, Tomarken, & Holtzbauer, 1982), they can maximize their performance if they keep records of successful execution of components of that performance. Related evidence from basic laboratory research also indicates that such positive self-monitoring of difficult tasks can sustain involvement or persistence in the task (see Kirschenbaum & Tomarken, 1982). Certainly these results suggest that high risk and sedentry adults should be taught to self-monitor positively when they begin their exercise and sport programs.

Environmental Management

Dishman's Chapter in this volume emphasizes that social-environmental factors can affect persistence in exercise programs. Degree and type of social support, whether the activity is social or solitary, and convenience factors all contribute to maintenance of exercise programs. The self-regulatory perspective merely argues that the individual can learn to shape his or her environment in a proactive fashion to maximize the probability of goal attainment.

It is also noteworthy that the type of external feedback provided to exercise and sport participants is another important environmental contributor to fitness outcomes. Extremely negativistic coaches need to be avoided and replaced by coaches, playing partners, and team members who provide ample support and encouragement (e.g., Smith, Small, & Curtis, 1979).

Generalization

Anti-sedentarianism, by definition, encourages very long-term, *chronic,* or lifestyle, changes. Maintenance of change in refractory behaviors, like exercising, seem to require the development of an "obsessive-compulsive style of self-regulation" (Kirschenbaum & Tomarken, 1982). That is, the evidence suggests that a great many factors can deter sustained self-regulated behavior change. In order to avoid self-regulatory failure, it seems necessary to self-monitor target behaviors continually, without letting emotional stressors, depressive or negativistic thinking, physiological pressures and other factors described elsewhere (Kirschenbaum, 1984b) dismantle sustained and systematic attention to target behaviors.

Research in sport psychology supports this conceptualization by showing that elite athletes often develop an obsessive-compulsive style of maintaining their efforts in their sports. Studies with gymnasts (Mahoney & Avener, 1977), golfers (Kirschenbaum & Bale, 1980), wrestlers (Gould, Weiss, & Weinberg, 1981; Highlen & Bennett, 1984), and divers (Highlen & Bennett, 1984) indicate that a variety of ritualistic behaviors and thoughts are associated with favorable performance outcomes. Mahoney and Avener (1977), for example, found that the frequency of thoughts about their sport in "everyday situations" correlated significantly with performance among elite gymnasts. Kirschenbaum and Bale (1980) established an even more direct connection. Better golf scores obtained by university-level golfers were positively correlated with the "obsessive" factor of Nideffer's (1976) Test Attentional and Interpersonal Style. In a more recent and larger scale study, Highlen and Bennett (1984) found that qualifiers for recent Canadian national wrestling and diving teams reported relatively high frequences of compulsive-like behaviors. These included withdrawal from others, frequent self-talk, and generally living a highly structured lifestyle, compared to similarly skilled athletes who failed to qualify for the national teams.

Unfortunately, it is far from clear how to help people develop obsessive-compulsive self-regulatory styles. This conceptualization does, however, suggest that relatively brief (acute) interventions and mass media campaigns should not be *expected* to produce substantial long-term change. Individual and small group interventions that are intensive, multi-component in focus, involving, and long-lasting appear warranted. For example, use of well-developed behavioral contracting could yield important, and as yet untapped, benefits (see Kirschenbaum & Flanery, 1983, 1984). Contracting is a flexible self-involving tool that people can implement largely on their own with brief consultation from others. Use of this procedure also helps assure that sustained self-monitoring will continue and it provides a forum for explicit goal-setting, planning, and environmental management. In addition, relapse prevention training (Marlatt & Gordon, 1980) could be utilized effectively in conjunction with behavioral contracting when individuals and small groups are the targets for intervention.

In sum, concepts and strategies of prevention appear useful when applied to the problem of sedentarianism are both important and attainable goals. Issues pertaining to the focus, timeframe, and target population must be considered when designing preventive interventions. Thus, certain programs that focus on environmental modification, as well as providing information, may produce some primary prevention benefits even when applied to organizations, communities, and societies. On the other hand, secondary prevention of sedentarianism with high risk and already somewhat sedentary adults probably requires multi-focused, intensive, and long-term (chronic) interventions targeted to individuals or groups. The latter efforts also must conceptualize the target of intervention as a refractory self-control problem. Principles and procedures developed to ameliorate such problems seem highly relevant, and worthy of explicit application, to anti-sedentarianism.

4

DEVELOPING AN ACTIVITY PLAN FOR IMPROVING HEALTH

William L. Haskell

INTRODUCTION

A wide variety of health and performance benefits have been attributed to the adoption of a physically active lifestyle. These benefits include both improvements in physical and psychological health status as well as enhanced physical and mental performance. Whereas a cause and effect relationship has been established between exercise and certain of these benefits, other potential benefits are supported only by associative or anecdotal data. Of the major claims for health, those with the greatest scientific basis are the contributions of exercise to maintenance of optimal body weight or composition and the normalization of fat and carbohydrate metabolism. Other benefits that have been reported in some circumstances include maintenance of bone mineral content with aging, the prevention or alleviation of low back pain syndrome, the prevention of coronary heart disease, reduction of elevated systemic arterial blood pressure and enhanced psychological status, including improved self image and confidence and decreased anxiety, depression and hostility.

There are a number of other disorders where if patients exercise they tend to show clinical improvement, but there is no evidence that exercise prevents such diseases. Included in this category are Type I diabetes, chronic obstructive lung disease (emphysema and bronchitis), renal failure, arthritis and various major psychological disorders. There is little, if any, data supporting the notion that exercise prevents any infectious disease or alters susceptibility to malignant neoplasm formation, and physically active people generally have a greater morbidity and mortality from accidents than would be expected if they remained sedentary.

Some of the research that has addressed the health and performance benefits of exercise also has attempted to determine the characteristics of the exercise and the exercise situation or environment required for the desired changes to occur. Most of this research has focused on the type, intensity and amount (duration X frequency) of exercise performed with the outcome variables most frequently being changes in aerobic capacity or adiposity. The dose-response relationship between increased exercise and other biologic variables has not been well established, while almost no systematic attention has been paid so far to the exercise characteristics that are required or are most effective in producing favorable psychological changes, including an increased ability to cope with mental stress.

The major objectives of this chapter are to review the scientific basis for designing a physical activity plan to improve general health, why and how exercise might be used as a stress coping maneuver and specific guidelines for designing and implementing a health oriented activity plan. The primary orientation of the material presented is to provide the information needed by clinicians or counselors to design and implement individualized health oriented activity plans for clients and to assist them with maintaining a more active lifestyle.

PHYSICAL FITNESS VERSUS HEALTH

Increases in physical working capacity or physical fitness often are equated inappropriately with improvements in health status or disease prevention. At times, this is a very important but difficult distinction to make: while a very high level of physical fitness usually requires good health (probably less for mental health), an improvement in physical fitness does not insure an increase in health or resistance to disease. For example, patients with disorders such as emphysema, hypertension or severe depression can significantly increase their working capacity through exercise training without necessarily changing the severity of their disease or their medical prognosis. Becoming more physically fit and improving health status are interrelated but not synonymous. Thus, when considering the dose of exercise required for improving health, including the ability to better cope with mental stress, care needs to be taken in extrapolating from investigations that have used measures of fitness as the only outcome.

It should be emphasized here that the only way to achieve a significant increase in physical fitness (physical working capacity) is through a systematic increase in habitual exercise (exercise training). This increase in capacity is an adaptative response by the body to the stress placed on various tissues and biologic functions by the increased metabolic or physical demands of the exercise. If the appropriate type of exercise is performed at the proper intensity, duration and frequency, sedentary individuals of all ages will achieve significant improvements in physical working capacity (American College of Sports Medicine, 1978). Following training, individuals are able to exercise at a greater intensity and for a longer duration than before, and they experience less fatigue at the same submaximal exercise. This increase in functional capacity is due primarily to enhanced metabolic capacity of skeletal muscle, increased capacity for substrate and oxygen delivery to the skeletal muscle by the cardiorespiratory system and changes in autonomic nervous system regulation during exercise.

WHAT EXERCISE STIMULI ARE REQUIRED TO IMPROVE HEALTH?

What has to occur when a person exercises so that the desired changes in health are produced? If exercise causes these benefits, then there needs to be some defined stimulus (or stimuli) that takes place as a result of participating in the exercise. Is the effect acute (during or immediately after exercise) or chronic (a delayed response or training effect)? Is it chemical, mechanical, situational, social or some combination? While a great deal of descriptive information exists on various training effects, very little is known about the controlling mechanisms or stimuli required to produce them.

For some health benefits, such as improved fat and carbohydrate metabolism and increased insulin sensitivity, the necessary stimulus appears to be similar to that required for the improvement in aerobic capacity: a sustained increase in the rate of energy expenditures by large skeletal muscles. This enhanced energy production during and following exercise increases the functioning of other biologic systems needed to support the raised metabolic rate and, with repeated stimulation, will increase capacity or efficiency. It is the adaptive response of these other systems, including the central nervous system, that appears to provide many of the physical health benefits of exercise. However, it is not yet clear whether it is simply the repeated acute effects of exercise, or a chronic training effect, that produces some of the health related benefits ascribed to aerobic-type training.

The stimulus for other health benefits is less well defined and may be related more to the physical stress placed on the muscles, connective tissue or skeleton. For instance, the retention of bone calcium through exercise following menopause may be the result of physical forces placed on the bone by weight bearing exercise. It is also possible that the enhanced metabolic rate associated with the increase in muscle mass is best achieved by the use of resistive exercise.

We know very little about the required stimuli for the various psychological benefits ascribed to exercise. Are the effects due to changes in biology resulting from the exercise itself, are they behavioral and due to the interaction between the exerciser and the exercising situation or are these effects due to some combined biobehavioral factors? Do some psychological effects require strictly a biologic stimulus such as an alteration in sympathetic nervous system activity, while others are dependent on a behavioral stimulus such as physical separation from the stress producing situation or the interaction with an exercise leader or other exercisers?

In coping with mental stress, what are the critical stimuli required of exercise for it to be an effective modality? From the little that seems to be

"Time out" Therapy

known about this issue, it appears that there may be multiple stimuli, some behavioral and some biologic. As Bahrke and Morgan (1978) have pointed out, exercise may be a useful stress coping mechanism for some people simply as "time out" therapy. Leisure time activity can be an effective way of physically and mentally separating oneself from stress producing situations at work or home. The physical separation plus pleasant surroundings, an enthusiastic exercise leader and sympathetic co-exercisers may be all that is required to decrease anxiety, hostility or depression: the actual exercise and its biologic effects may be secondary. Added to this possibility are the diversionary effects of competition with oneself to do better or to do well (or win) when competing with others along with the stimulus of excitement or risk of some activities. The stress produced by a failing business or unmanageable teenager is at least temporarily discarded when a 55 year old club tennis player is playing the last set in the finals of a local masters tournament or when an alpine skier plunges down 2,000 feet through two feet of new Utah powder.

Added to the situational or behavioral stimuli for enhanced psychological status, including enhanced capacity to cope with mental stress, may be biologic stimuli such as altered central nervous system/hormonal regulation (Cousineau, Ferguson & deChamplain, 1977), improved exercise capacity (endurance, strength, flexibility) and changes in appearance (weight loss, increased muscle tone and mass). If a person can work harder and longer at a physical task with less fatigue, can he/she cope better with mental stress? The same question can be asked regarding appearance: do people who feel better about looking better (usually meaning younger) cope better with stressful situations?

Defining the required stimulus for the desired training effect is crucial to developing an effective activity plan. Unless some general idea regarding the nature of the stimuli is known, it is not possible to target an activity plan to meet the specific goal of stress reduction. If the primary stimulus is situational (e.g., "time out") then the diversity of activity plans recommended may be substantial and designed based on an entirely different set of criteria than if the stimulus is tied to a large and sustained rise in circulating catecholamines or endorphins which can be obtained only by exercises that meet very specific criteria.

PRINCIPLES OF EXERCISE TRAINING

There are three principles or concepts that apply to exercise training, the knowledge of which can be extremely valuable in helping clients understand how the health benefits of exercise are achieved. The application of these principles form the biologic basis for developing an individualized activity plan. While we have some understanding of how these concepts apply to training effects, like improved cardiovascular and metabolic capacity, we presently have access to very little data on their application to the specific psychological benefits of exercise.

Overload: The principle of overload is the key to nearly all of the physical performance and health benefits produced by exercise training. Overload means that the body responds to an increase in activity by a combination or series of adaptations. Even a slight increase in the intensity or amount of exercise over what is usually performed will make new demands on the various tissues or systems in the body, and they respond to this demand by enhancing their capacity or efficiency. This is the basis for the advice that when starting an exercise program, simply do more today than you did yesterday, and then do slightly more tomorrow. Thus, exercise training effects are nothing more than the body's attempt to adjust to the new demands or stresses. The characteristics of the adaptations the body will make to this new exercise demand will depend on the type of exercise, its intensity and its amount.

The effects of overload may not be linear and are not similar in magnitude for all benefits. Absolute thresholds have been difficult to establish but some criteria have been recommended. For example, changes in aerobic capacity appear to be most effectively produced (improvement/effort) when previously sedentary individuals exercise at 50% to 80% of their aerobic capacity: at lower intensities and above the dose response curve tends to be relatively flat. This intensity applies when exercise is performed for more than 10 minutes per session for two or more sessions per week (American College of Sports Medicine, 1978).

The magnitude of the overload required to produce a beneficial effect will depend on the person's recent activity status. While this concept especially applies to the intensity of exercise, it also seems to apply to the total amount of exercise performed. Very inactive people tend to gain relatively greater biologic benefit from very modest amounts of exercise (Badenhop, Cleary, Schaal, Fox, & Bartels, 1983). Also, complete inactivity, such as bed rest, rapidly decreases physical working capacity, glucose tolerance and high density lipoprotein cholesterol with most of these changes reversible with the return of usual activity patterns.

Progression: The principle of progression simply means that in order for a person to continue to experience improvement as a result of exercise, the increased exercise demand (overload) needs to be applied in small increments. After a few days or weeks of exercising at a set amount or intensity, the body has adapted to those demands and new adaptations will occur only when exercise is increased by a small amount. If an individual does not try to progress too quickly, the adaptations the body makes to increased demands are positive. Whereas if one attempts to progress too rapidly, there is the tendency to produce unnecessary fatigue, soreness and tissue injury or damage. Most people want to try and improve too quickly and this lack of patience will lead to frustration, unnecessary fatigue and possible injury. Also, it is important to realize that not everyone will progress at the same rate. Some people will take longer and progress more slowly. This may be due to their basic constitution or heredity, past exercise patterns, or current health status. For example, being substantially overweight or a heavy cigarette smoker may result in a slower rate of progression.

Specificity: The concept of specificity implies that adaptations will occur only in those tissues or body systems that experience increased demands or "overload" during exercise. For example, if the goal is to increase stamina, then activity has to be performed that puts demands on the oxygen transport and metabolic functions of the body since they are what primarily limits stamina in the healthy person. If the goal is to increase strength of the legs, then it is necessary to perform resistive exercise with those muscles. Exercising the arms is not an effective way to increase the capacity of the legs and vice versa. Lifting heavy weight will not increase cardiovascular endurance capacity nor will jogging increase the muscle tone of the arms. Thus, specificity not only applies to parts of the body, but also to types of changes (endurance, strength, flexibility, weight loss, etc.) that are desired from the exercise program. Due to specificity, it is necessary to select the right exercise to meet the specific goals of the client, and as the goals change the activities performed may need to be changed as well. Specificity means that many effects of different types of exercise are not interchangeable.

The concept of specificity can only be applied in the design of an activity plan when the stimulus needed to produce the desired effect is known. The required stimuli have not been established for many of the psychological or behavioral benefits attributed to exercise, thus making it impossible to apply specificity in a precise way in designing exercise programs to prevent or alleviate mental stress. The stimuli for stress reduction may vary depending on the individual as well as the characteristics of the stress. Preliminary evidence indicates that more vigorous aerobic type exercise may be more effective in relieving stress (Morgan, 1979), but this has not been the case in all situations (Barhke & Morgan, 1978).

THE DOSE RESPONSE RELATIONSHIP

A question frequently asked by the exerciser and nonexerciser alike, is how much exercise do I need to become fit or insure good health? Obviously, the correct answer to such a question will depend on the specific goals of the individual and certain personal characteristics such as age, sex, heredity, health status and recent activity habits. As discussed previously, quite precise answers can be given to this dose-response question for improving aerobic capacity or muscular strength or decreasing body weight. But for other health benefits, especially the psychological components, precise dose-response or threshold data are not available.

An example of the exercise and health dose-response data is the apparent relationship between habitual activity and coronary heart disease risk. The results of various studies that have related on-the-job or leisure-time activity levels to the incidence of coronary heart disease indicate that a daily energy expenditure of 200 to 400 kilocalories per day of leisure-time activity at moderate intensity is associated with a lower risk of heart attack (Table 1).

A reduction in risk appears to begin to occur with relatively small amounts of exercise with risk decreasing as exercise increases up to a maximum threshold of 3000 kilocalories per week. Paffenbarger, Wing and Hyde (1978) demonstrated that as Harvard Alumni increased their leisure-time activity from 500 kilocalories per week, there was a continuing decrease in heart attack rate up to an energy expenditure of 2000 to 3000 per week, above which no further benefit was observed. Similar results indicating that much of the health benefit is associated with getting people who are doing nothing to do something as compared to getting already active people to do more, have been observed by other investigators (Shapiro, Weinblatt, Frank, & Sager, 1969; Salonen, Puska, & Tuomilehto, 1982).

With respect to dose-response, there are several issues that seem important to consider in not only designing an activity plan, but also in attempting to maintain long-term adherence. First is the issue that many health benefits of exercise, including some of the important psychological benefits, might be

TABLE 1 Physical activity level (kilocalories) associated with a reduced risk of coronary heart disease

Study	Kilocalories		Type of activity
	Rate/min*	Total/day*	
Job-related activity			
North Dakota-USA	5–8	300–600	Farming & laboring
Evans County-USA	3–7.5	400–500	Farming & laboring
Railroad-USA	5–8	350–600	Walking, climbing, hanging
Health Insurance Clients-USA	4–8	300–500	Walking, lifting, carrying
Longshoremen-USA	5.2–7.5	810	Cargo handlers
Non-job activity			
Civil Servants-Eng.	4–7	100–140	Walking 5 days/week
Health Insurance Clients-USA	4–12	250–500	Walking, recreation, home activity
College Graduates-USA	3–12	250–350	Walking, stair climbing, sports
Civil Servants-Eng.	7.5	225	Recreation, home activity

Note: Adapted from Haskell, W. L.: Cardiovascular Benefits and Risks of Exercise, in Strauss, R. H. (ed.): *Sports Medicine.* W. B. Saunders Company, 1984.

  *Estimated kilocalorie per minute expenditure for 70 kilogram man.

  **Estimated difference in total kilocalories per day expenditure between the least active and more active subjects.

achievable by relatively small but very frequent increases in activity by sedentary people. This concept is contrary to that promoted by many health or fitness professionals and overlooked by most of the "Pepsi Generation" commercials promoting exercise (and their product) through mass media. This image that high level exercise is required in order to gain health benefits may be a major deterrent to many sedentary middle-age or older individuals initiating any kind of exercise program. The tendency has been to use the dose of exercise required to increase aerobic capacity as the "gold standard" for all health benefits as well. Activity programs that have not significantly increased aerobic capacity within 8 to 16 weeks have been considered of no or little value. Many health benefits appear to accrue to the previously sedentary adult as a result of only modest increases in activity if performed on a very frequent basis. Small amounts of exercise daily can lead to significant weight loss if caloric intake remains constant, blood clotting and fibrinolysis may be enhanced, bone mineral content retained in the elderly and possibly enhanced psychological status. There is a need for thorough investigations of the potential health benefits of relatively low intensity, large muscle, dynamic exercise. If it can be shown to be beneficial, it may be possible to get many sedentary adults who will not perform the more vigorous activity frequently promoted to perform low intensity exercise.

The second issue is what seems to be the highly consistent finding from many studies that the adequate activity dose to produce many of the established biologic benefits of exercise (some possibly the basis for psychological benefits as well) is an energy expenditure of somewhere around 300 kilocalories per exercise session (4 kilocalories per kilogram body weight to be more precise), performed using large muscles in a rhythmical fashion, at a moderate intensity relative to the individual's aerobic capacity and on the basis of every two to three days. This dose has been shown consistently to improve aerobic capacity and contribute to a reduction in body weight (American College of Sports Medicine, 1978), enhance insulin sensitivity (Soman, Veikko, Deibert, Felig, & DeFronzo, 1979), improve plasma lipoprotein profiles (Wood, Haskell, Blair, Ho, Williams, & Farquhar, 1983) and provide psychological benefit (Morgan, 1979). Exercise of a lesser dose provides some of these benefits but the changes are less consistent and are of smaller magnitude, whereas exercise of a substantially greater dose may provide additional benefits or the same benefits more rapidly. These benefits, though, are not well defined and with this greater exercise dosage comes the increased risk of exercise induced or aggrevated injury.

CHARACTERISTICS OF ACTIVITY TO PROMOTE HEALTH

An individualized activity plan can be described by the type, intensity, duration and frequency of the exercise to be performed. The specifics for each of these characteristics should depend on the individual's goals, exercise capacity, interests, skills and exercise opportunities (schedule, facilities, equipment, partners, competitors, etc.). Characteristics of the plan should change depending on increases in exercise capacity, development of new skills or interests and changes in opportunities (change of season, new facilities, new acquaintances). For individuals who have not had any exercise experience, the participation for several months in a supervised exercise program conducted by a knowledgeable exercise leader or specialist can be of substantial value in selecting the appropriate exercise, setting the proper intensity and developing the proper technique or skills.

Exercise Type

The type of exercise that provides the greatest health benefits and permits the greatest increase in energy expenditure with the least fatigue consists of performing rhythmical contractions of large muscles to move the body over a distance or against gravity. Such exercise frequently is referred to as being endurance or "aerobic" since, if it is performed at an intensity that is moderate relative to an individual's capacity and most of the resynthesis of high energy compounds in the muscle takes place in the presence of oxygen. Included in this type of exercise is walking, hiking, jogging or running, cycling, cross-country skiing, swimming, active games and sports, selected calisthenics and vigorous at-home or on-the-job chores. While very specific activities are required when training for competition in many athletic events, for health purposes, any exercise of this type seems to be beneficial if performed long and frequently enough at the proper intensity.

Based on the limited data available, if the psychological benefits of exercise have a biochemical basis, then it is sustained aerobic exercise that most likely will provide the necessary stimulus. During and following such exercise, there is a large rise in cathecholamine production which may signal changes in central nervous system regulation which allow for the more effective coping with mental stress. For example, it has been demonstrated that plasma catecholamine concentrations at a constant exercise intensity are lower following exercise training (Cousineau, Ferguson, & deChamplain, 1977) and that lymphocyte beta receptor activity is reduced as a result of endurance exercise training (Gordon, Savin, Bristow, & Haskell, 1983). Also, an increase in circulating beta endorphin concentrations appears to occur with endurance-type exercise (Carr, Bullen, & Skrinar, 1981), although the clinical meaning of which is not understood.

This dynamic exercise is in contrast to static or heavy resistance exercise that produces primarily a pressure load rather than a volume load on the cardiovascular system which results in very rapid muscle fatigue at relatively low rates of energy expenditure and primarily produces local muscle rather than more general systemic adaptations. Heavy resistance exercise is useful for the development of muscle strength and muscle tone or mass (which can be important psychologically for some men and an increasing number of women) and is useful in rehabilitation following musculo-skeletal injury. For some individuals, self image and confidence seems to be enhanced by this type of exercise. Appendix I contains a comprehensive listing of activities, their relative contribution to the development of various components of physical fitness and stress management and their degree of risk or hazard. This list can be used with clients to select appropriate activities when designing their exercise plan.

Exercise Intensity

The exercise induced biologic changes that contribute to health are achieved when the exercise intensity is somewhat greater than that usually performed by the individual. This increase in intensity causes adaptations that allow the metabolic needs of the muscles being exercised to be more readily met. While exercise intensities that are even slightly greater than that usually performed will promote changes, the usual recommendation is that exercise for optimizing health should be performed at 50 to 75 percent of the individual's oxygen transport capacity or at 60 to 85 percent of maximum achievable heart rate during exercise (see Figure 1).

Using these guidelines, exercise training heart rates for individuals 30 years of age would range from 114 to 162 beats per minute, whereas at age 60, the range would be from 96 to 137 beats per minute (based on the calculation that maximal exercise heart rate is approximately 220—age in years). For most people, this recommendation produces a substantial intensity overload since they usually do not exercise at more than about 40 percent of their aerobic capacity during everyday activities.

Exercise Amount

The exercise duration to be recommended will depend on the person's health or fitness goals and exercise capacity as well as on the type of exercise to be performed. One interpretation of the data available on exercise and health is

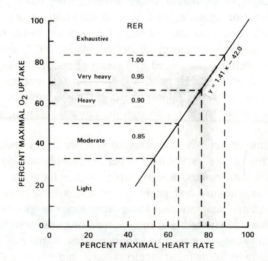

FIGURE 1

that people who do even a small amount of exercise on a regular basis are better off than those that do almost nothing. A reasonable goal seems to be an energy expenditure over usual activities of approximately 300 kilocalories per session with a frequency of at least every two to three days. Most clinically healthy adults have the capacity to expend from 400 to 700 kilocalories per hour while performing aerobic, large-muscle activity of a moderate intensity. Thus, they can expend 300 kilocalories in 25 to 45 minutes. Activities meeting this goal include walking or jogging 4 kilometers, cycling or swimming for 20 minutes or playing several sets of tennis in 45 minutes. Whereas lower intensity exercise such as walking or gardening will not produce a large increase in exercise capacity, if performed for longer periods and more frequently, it seems to provide many of the physical health benefits derived from more vigorous exercise (e.g., facilitates weight control, bone mineral retention and glucose tolerance).

Designing an Activity Plan to Improve Health

The results of many of the studies cited in the prior sections of this report tend to have a common theme: from a health perspective, more active people tend to do better physically and mentally than their very sedentary counterparts and the type and the amount of exercise required to attain many of these benefits is achievable by most motivated adults. Since the health benefits are diverse, and substantial variation exists among adults regarding their exercise capacity, interests, skills and accessability, an individualized activity plan or exercise prescription needs to be developed in order to maximize the likelihood of a successful outcome.

Many of the concepts and procedures that serve as the basis for exercise training used to prepare for athletic competition have been applied to the designing of activity plans for health improvement. While some of these ideas and methods have been proven to be quite transferable, others are not only inappropriate but actually may be misleading or contraindicated. For example, while the idea of "no pain, no gain" may be needed for achieving peak athletic performance, such an approach is not needed and may be detrimental in using exercise to maintain health or prevent disease.

Since the stimuli required of exercise to increase a person's ability to cope with mental stress or the dose-response relationship between exercise and stress reduction has not been adequately defined, the design of an activity plan to reduce stress has to be based, at least in part, on other exercise—health/fitness relationships and certain assumptions.

Flexibility in developing the exercise plan needs to be retained since the most important consideration is that the plan will lead to an increase in activity by the client and that this increase will result in a permanent change. A great plan is no good unless the client increases his/her activity in a manner that produces the desired results.

The first objective is to try and establish clear goals, both short and long range. They should be quite explicit and ideally be put in writing. These goals can be defined either as outcomes (weight loss of 10 pounds) or of actions (jog for 30 minutes 3 times per week). Even though many clients are exercising for health reasons, it is not possible for them to quantify their goals other than in terms of actions or improved physical working capacity (how does the client quantify the goal of a better stress coping capacity?). Goals need to be periodically reassessed with a change towards maintenance from improvement as the program progresses.

Once the goals have been established, the specifics of the activity plan need to be defined. Instead of selecting a single activity around which the success of the plan revolves, have the client establish a period of time to exercise a certain number of days per week and then fill that time with whatever appropriate exercise is available (See Appendix I for exercise selection). For example, the client may set his target at 20 minutes per day on weekdays and 40 minutes on one weekend day. During weekdays the activity may consist of walking or stationary cycling and on weekends it may involve swimming or tennis. On the other hand, some people like, and are more successful at, a highly regimented program of the very same activity at the very same time each day (however, this is usually the already dedicated exerciser).

In an attempt to have the client use exercise as a stress management tool, a location away from stress producing situations should be selected (I believe outdoors is highly preferable), the type of exercise should be aerobic, the intensity moderate (initially at 50 to 60% of aerobic capacity), the duration for at least 30 minutes and the frequency at least every other day. Ideally, the exercise should be supervised (at least for some of the sessions) and if in a group setting, each participant should be allowed to exercise at his/her own pace. *Relaxation techniques should be taught as an integral part of the plan and practiced at the end of every activity session.*

In addition to the specific time set aside for exercise training, each client should have recommendations on how to increase activity throughout the remainder of the day as part of his/her exercise plan. How to best achieve this goal has not been established even though it is frequently suggested by health counselors. Here, the major idea is to get previously sedentary people thinking of themselves as exercisers and to be constantly looking for opportunities to exercise rather than avoiding it.

In addition to endurance-type activities, some exercises which maintain or develop muscle strength and flexibility of joints need to be included as a part of the activity plan. These activities contribute to a retention of lean body mass, may help protect against injury and contribute to the prevention of low back pain. Only a few minutes of these exercises per day are required to achieve significant increases in strength and flexibility, and they can be performed before or after the endurance exercise or at a separate time.

EXERCISE SAFETY

When recommending exercise for health promotion, one does battle with the proverbial two-edged sword. Inappropriate exercise can literally pose dangers to limbs and life. The most commonly encountered problem is that of musculoskeletal discomfort or injury due to overuse or trauma. Of more severe consequences, but much less frequent, is the precipitation of a major cardiac arrest. However, the likelihood is remote that exercise will cause such a cardiac event in individuals without significant underlying cardiac disease.

Orthopedic injuries occur most often during health oriented exercise as a result of the added weight bearing stress on feet, ankles, legs, knees and lower back associated with jogging, running and racket sports. Most of these injuries are due to irritations of tendons, ligaments, bones and sometimes muscles. There is a wide range of susceptibility to such injuries and it is difficult to predict who will or will not have problems as the intensity and amount of exercise performed increases. Risk become greater with advancing age, history of previous injury, overuse and substantial obesity. Preventive procedures include the use of non-weight bearing activities such as swimming, stationary cycling or rowing and substituting brisk walking or hiking for jogging. If possible, exercise should be performed on soft surfaces and jumping type activities, including aerobic dancing on hard floors, may need to be avoided. Well constructed athletic or running shoes with thick shock absorbing soles, raised heels and arch supports are a good investment for the serious exerciser. It is important to begin a new program very slowly (progression) to allow the body's support structures adequate time to accommodate to the new stress being placed on them (every other day activity rather than daily activity may be preferred for people who are injury prone). When problems do develop, it is important to relieve the stress by decreasing the intensity or amount of activity, switching to an alternative exercise or resting and applying appropriate therapy. Clients should be instructed to listen to "body signals" and when overuse pain persists, it is time to back off or change activities.

Most cardiac events can be prevented if individuals remain under good general medical care (periodic evaluations and appropriate therapy when indicated), control major cardiac risk factors, learn the proper skills for health-oriented exercise, use this knowledge in carrying out a program of regular exercise and take heed of "body signals" that indicate the exercise plan should be modified or medical attention sought. Proper medical clearance, individualized program planning and implementation and personal monitoring are the keys to safe exercise.

There are many other health risks of exercise but these usually are limited to individuals with established disease (e.g., diabetes, heart disease, chronic obstructive lung disease, asthma or renal failure) or occur with very extended or competitive exercise. The most important of these risks is the development of severe heat injury. The total prevention of these injuries cannot be achieved if adults are to increase their exercise, but the risks can be reduced by proper medical evaluation, individualized activity planning, and improved public education.

CONCLUSIONS

It has been well documented that appropriate exercise can make a substantial contribution to a comprehensive program of both physical and mental health improvement. Psychological benefits include reductions in anxiety, hostility and depression and probably an enhanced capacity for coping with mental stress. More research is required to determine the many specifics regarding the cause-effect relationship between increased exercise and improved psychological status. Important topics include: what type of exercise and how much is needed to produce clinically significant benefits, what is the required stimulus for each of the effects (behavioral versus biological) and how can clients be identified who will be helped by exercise as well as those who need some other form of therapy.

The exercise required to achieve many of the health benefits is well within the capacity of most healthy adults. Dynamic exercise involving large muscle groups performed at moderate intensity appears to contribute the most to both physical and mental health status with the major stimulus for improvement being a sustained increase in energy expenditure. Initial goals should be to increase activity level so that an additional 150 to 200 kilocalories are expended per session with the longer term goal being an activity plan that requires an expenditure of 300 kilocalories at a moderate intensity at least every other day.

The greatest success in maintaining health-oriented exercise is obtained with individually designed programs that consider personal interests, skills and exercise opportunities as well as goals and exercise capacity. Time should be set aside at least every other day for exercise and it should be filled with one of several appropriate activities rather than selecting a single exercise as the only basis for increasing activity level. The activity generally should be convenient to perform, fit within the person's general lifestyle and be enjoyable. For the purpose of using exercise to help manage stress, it should be combined with other behavioral techniques directed at the same goal.

APPENDIX I Benefits and hazards of various activities

Activity or exercise	METs[1]	KCAL per hr[2]	Cardio-respiratory endurance	Muscle strength, power & endurance	Coordination, balance & grace	Flexibility & agility	Stress management/diversion[3]	Social opportunities	Injury hazard problems[4]
Archery	2–3	150–250	+walking	+++arms, shoulders	+++eyes, arms	+	++	++ – +++	Small, if care taken
Backpacking	3–8	250–600	++walking +++climbing	++	+	+ – +++	+	+++	Sprains, back strain
Badminton									
Social doubles	3–4	250–300	+	+	+++	+++	++	++++	++
Social singles	6	450	++	+	+++	+++	++	+++	±
Compet. singles	8–10	600–750	+++ – +++++	++	++++	++++	+++	++	±
Baseball or softball									
Except pitcher	2–3	150–250	±	+	+	+	Stressful waiting	+++	Hit by ball, bat; sliding trauma; sprains
Pitcher	6	450	++	++	+++	++	++	+++	
Basketball	4–10	300–750	++++	+++	++++	++++	+++	+++	Collision injuries; knees, ankles back
Bicycling (on level)									
5 mph	3	250	+	±legs	++	±	stressful in traffic; otherwise +++	+++	Traffic hazards and spills
10 mph	6	450	++	++	++	±		++	
13 mph	9	650	+++ – +++++	+++	++	+	+++	+	
Boardsailing	3–8	250–600	++ – +++	++ – +++++	+++ – +++++	+++	+++	++	Bruises; hypothermia
Bowling	1½–3	100–225	little	little	++	++	±	++++	Low
Calisthenics	2–8	150–600	++ – +++++	+ for most +++ for some	++ – +++	++++ if varied	++	++	Few, with good warm-ups

APPENDIX I Benefits and hazards of various activities (*Continued*)

Activity or exercise	METs[1]	KCAL per hr[2]	Cardio-respiratory endurance	Muscle strength, power & endurance	Coordination, balance & grace	flexibility & agility	Stress management/ diversion[3]	Social opportunities	Injury hazard problems[4]
Canoeing									
flat water	2–8	150–600	++ – +++	+++	++	++	+++	+++	Drowning;
white water	5–10	400–750	+++ – +++++	++++	++++	++++	++++	++ – ++++	Hypothermia
Dancing									
Ballet & Modern	4–9+	300–700+	+++ – +++++	++ – ++++	++++	++++	+++	+++	Sprains, tears; strains
Vigorous Ballroom	3–8+	250–600	++ – +++	++	+++	+++	+++ if relaxed	++++	Few
Folk & Square	3–8+	250–600+	++ – +++	+++	+++	++	+++ if relaxed	++++	Few
"Aerobic"	5–9	300–700	+++ – +++++	+++	+++ – +++++	+++ – +++++	++++	++++	Rare men still reluctant
Fencing	6–9	450–700	+++	+++	++++	++++	+++	++	Considerable, if guards defective
Fishing									
Casting	2–3	150–250	little	–	+	++	+++	++	Fish hook in eyes; drowning; and hypothermia
Waling with waders	4–6	300–500	++	+	++	++	+++	++	
Football (while active)	6–9	450–700	++	+++	++	+++	Diverting	+++	+++
Gardening	2–8	150–600	++	++	+	+++	+++	++	Few
Golf	2–4	150–300	++ walking	±	++ highly specific	+++ highly specific	++ if relaxed	+++ – ++++	Hit by ball or club
Gymnastics	3–5	250–400	++ – +++++	++++ – +++++	++++	++++	+++	++	Occasional
Handball	6–10	450–750	+++ – +++++	+++	++++	+++	+++	++	Sprains, muscle tear
Hockey									
Field	8–10	600–750	+++	++	++	+++	+++	+++	Some
Ice	8–10	600–750	+++	++	++	++	+++	+++	More

Isometrics	2-5	150-400	+	up to ++++	little	+ – ++	±	+	Few
Isotonics	2-10+	150-800	+++	++	++	+++	++ – +++	++	Few
Jogging (see Running)									
Karate/Judo	6-10+	450-800+	+++ – +++++	++ – +++	++++	++++	Diverting & stressful	up to ++++	Contact injuries
Kayaking (see Canoeing)									
Mountain-climbing	6-8	450-800	+++	+++ – +++++	++	+++	Can be stressful	++	Falling rocks; avalanches
Mowing									
Pushing Power	3-4	250-300	+	++	little	little	little	little	Considerable
Pushing Hand	6-8	450-600	+++	+	little	little	little	little	Few
Paddleball	4-8	300-600	+++ – +++++	+++	+++	+++++	+++	+++	Eye injury
Platform Tennis									
Ping Pong (Table Tennis)	4-6	300-450	+++	++	+++	+++	+++	+++	Few
Racquetball	6-10	450-750	++++	+	+++	++++	+++	+++	Eye, racquet injuries
Raking Leaves	3-5	250-400	++	+++	+	++	++	+	Few
Riding Horseback	2-5	150-400	+ – +++	++	++	++	++	++	++
Rope Skipping	8-12	600-900	++++	+ – ++	+++	+++	+++	++	++
Rowing									
2 mph	3	250	+	+++	++	++	+++	+++	Upsets; hypothermia
4 mph	7	500	++	++	++	++	+++	+	
6 mph	12	900	++++	+++	++	++	+++	–	
Rugby	6-8	450-600	+++	++++	+	++	++	+++	Lacerations; bruises
Running & Jogging									
5 mph	7-8	500-600	+++	+++	little	little	+	++	Hit by autos; sprains
7 mph	12	800	++++	++	little	little	++	+	
9 mph	15	1100	++++	+++	little	little	+	+	
Sailing									
Crew	2-4	150-300	++	++++	+++	+++	+++	+++	Overboard hazards
Skipper	1-3	75-200	–	+++	+	+	++	++	

APPENDIX I Benefits and hazards of various activities *(Continued)*

Activity or exercise	METs[1]	KCAL per hr[2]	Cardio-respiratory endurance	Muscle strength, power & endurance	Coordination, balance & grace	Flexibility & agility	Stress management/diversion[3]	Social opportunities	Injury hazard problems[4]
Hand Sawing Hardwood	6-8	450-600	+++	+++	little	little	+	±	Cuts
Sexual Intercourse	5-8	400-600	. . Usually too brief . . .	too brief . . .	unlikely	++	++ − +++	?	Too macho or "conquest coronary"
Shoveling	5-9	400-700	++ − +++++	+++ − +++++	+	++	+++	±	Backstrain
Skating	4-10+	300-800+	++ − +++++	+++ − +++++	++++	+++	+++	++++	Falls; cuts
Skiing Cross country	5-12+	400-900+	++ − +++++	+++ − +++++	+++	+++	++++	+++	Few strains,
Downhill	4-10+	300-800+	++ − +++	+++ − +++++	++++	++++	++++	+++	fractures
Skin Diving	6-10	450-750	+++	+++	+	++	+++	+	Drowning; sharks; hypothermia
Soccer	8-10+	600-750+	+++ − +++	+++	++++	+++	+++	++	Collisions
Squash	8-10+	600-750	++++	+++	++++	++++	++++	++	Eye injuries; collisions
Surfing	4-7	300-500	++	+++	++++	++++	+++	++	Coral cuts
Swimming	4-10+	300-750	++++	+++	++	++	+++ one of best	+++	Drowning; hypothermia
Tennis	4-10	300-750	++ − +++++	+++	++++	+++	++	++++	Eye injuries; sunburn; sprains
Volleyball	4-7	300-500	++ − +++	++	+++	+++	++	++++	Sprains, collisions
Walking (on level) 2 mph 3 kph	2	150	+	±	±	little	+++	+++	Minimal
5 kph 4 mph	3+	250	++	+	+	little	+++	++	Minimal

54

Activity	METs	Kcal/hr							Injury & Hazard
6.5 kph	5-6	400-500	+++	++	++	++	+++	+	Low
(stairs/hills)	7-12+	500-900	+++	+++	++	++	++	++	Low
Waterskiing	4-8	300-600	+ - ++	+++	++	++	exciting	++	Propeller cuts; back strain
Weightlifting	3-6	250-450	+	++++	++	+	stressful	+	High blood pressure dropped weights
Windsurfing (see Boardsailing)									
Woodsplitting	2-6+	150-500	++ - +++	+++	+++	++	+++	+	Eye and foot injuries
Yoga	1-4	75-300	little	little	variable	up to ++++	may be excellent	+++	Few

Note: Reproduced with permission of Samuel M. Fox III, M.D., Preventive Cardiology Programs, Georgetown University Medical Center.

1) METs = Multiples of resting metabolic rate—when sitting. The range reflects the varying intensity, from the leisurely or recreational pace to the competitive or frenetic, that can be involved.

2) Kilocalories per hour—based on a 70 kg (154 lbs) weight. A 10% increase or decrease can be applied for each 7 kg (15 lbs) over or under 70 kg, respectively.

3) Stress management may operate by either of at least two mechanisms or both: a) diversion—making it difficult to continue about previous worries; b) through high level metabolic and muscular activity reduce chronic muscle tension and enhance sleep, rest and relaxation. Some activities such as karate and waterskiing may be "stressful" due to the excitement involved, but provide good recovery relaxation.

4) Injury & Hazard. Most hazards can be avoided with care and appropriate stretching; warming up and cooling down can help reduce strains, tears, and joint irritations that otherwise make some activities painful.

5

EXERCISE ADHERENCE AND HABITUAL PHYSICAL ACTIVITY

Rod K. Dishman

INTRODUCTION

There is an emerging consensus within exercise science, health psychology, behavioral medicine, and preventive medicine that the prediction and control of exercise behavior represents an important objective for the health sciences and professions (Dishman, 1982a; Martin & Dubbert, 1982; Oldridge, 1982). While other chapters in this volume address the validity of this view, the current chapter will involve an attempt to characterize the state of understanding about behavioral influences associated with programmatic exercise. The focus will be on problems of exercise adherence (Morgan, 1977), but these will be defined within a broader perspective of habitual physical activity. Because research on exercise behavior has collectively emanated from applied or pragmatic questions rather than from theory, the goal of this chapter will be to conceptualize major findings and methodological issues that appear to offer promise for directing research and clinical application. This will hopefully facilitate scholarly evaluations of what is now known, application to some practical advantage, and provoke hypotheses for evaluating and refining current models of exercise behavior. Earlier reviews have dealt with physical activity involvement (Morgan, 1977; Wankel, 1981), compliance in cardiac rehabilitation (Oldridge, 1982), obesity (Brownell & Stunkard, 1980), and adult fitness programs (Franklin, 1984; Sherpard, 1979). There have also been overviews of behavior management techniques applied to exercise (Epstein & Wing, 1980; Martin & Dubbert, 1984), as well as conceptual analyses of the exercise adherence literature (Dishman, 1982a, 1982b, 1984; Martin & Dubbert, 1982a, 1982b).

The timeliness of a state-of-the-art synopsis in exercise adherence seems reinforced by its recent inclusion as a definition area by the Behavioral Epidemiology and Evaluation Branch of the Public Health Service. On the other hand, a recent and comprehensive discussion of behavioral interventions and compliance to treatment regimes did not include exercise or physical activity (Benfari, Eaker, & Stoll, 1981).

SCOPE OF THE PROBLEM

Despite reports that 1) 30 million adults are runners or joggers in the United States (American Running & Fitness Association, 1981), 2) that weight training has recently surpassed running to become the seventh most popular form of recreation (Neilsen, 1983), and 3) that there is widespread use of community sport facilities (Thomas, Lee, Franks, & Paffenbarger, 1981), it has been estimated that two-thirds of American adults do not exercise regularly (Harris, 1978; Gallup, 1985) and 45% do not exercise at all (Clarke, 1974; Gallup, 1984). Among individuals who voluntarily enter a supervised exercise program by physician referral or self-selection, it is common to observe a 50% dropout within six-months (Dishman, 1982; Morgan, 1977), and dropout curves are typically described by a negative acceleration up to this point. These curves usually plateau at 12 to 24 months (Carmody, Senner, Malinow, & Matarazzo, 1980; Morgan, 1977; Oldridge, 1982) and a small, gradual attrition occurs thereafter. There has been a lack of follow-up on adherents and dropouts once these studies have been completed. Dropout rates have ranged from a low of 11% for one year (Greist, Klein, Eischens, Faris, Gurman, & Morgan, 1979), to a high of 87% (Kentala, 1972).

Because health-related exercise patterns appear to mirror recidivism rates for several abusive behaviors including smoking, excess weight, and drug dependence (Morgan, 1977), it has been suggested that the decision to discontinue an exercise program parallels the general problem of medical compliance (Dishman, 1982) and that a physically active lifestyle may be a fundamental component of behavioral health (Belloc & Breslow, 1972; Breslow & Enstrom, 1980). The U.S. Public Health Service Centers for Disease Control have estimated that one-half the mortality for the ten leading causes of death in the United States is strongly linked to habitual behaviors, and reports by the Surgeon General (Califano, 1979) and the Institute of Medicine (Hamburg, 1982) include physical inactivity among major health risk behaviors. As part of a public health promotion strategy, the United States Department of Health and Human Services (1982) and the American Medical Association (1983) recently endorsed the type of exercise guidelines proposed earlier by the American College of Sports Medicine (1978) to insure gains in cardiopulmonary and neuromuscular fitness. Surveys of primary care physicians and psychiatrists confirm that exercise is a common prescription for clinical disorders including moderate depression, anxiety, tension, cardiovascular and pulmonary diseases, diabetes, low back disorder, and drug dependence (Dishman, 1985). There also appears to be a proliferation of health-related fitness programs in corporate (Fielding, 1982), community (Meyer, Nash, McAlister, Maccoby, & Farquhar, 1980), and public school (Blair, Falls, & Pate, 1983) settings in addition to the commercial sector. The health-exercise-adherence triad may be a particularly important concern for health policy in public education, because some of the CHD risk factors known to be responsive to exercise have been found in adolescents (Wilmore, Constable, Sanforth, Tsao, Rotkis, Paicios, Mattern, & Ewy, 1982).

While estimates of the health, fitness and fiscal impact of these programs are beginning to appear in research journals (e.g., Pomerleau, 1983; Thomas, Lee, Franks, & Paffenbarger, 1981), their behavioral impact has not been studied systematically. It is estimated, however, that only 20% of employees will participate in occupational exercise programs (Shephard, Morgan, Finucane, & Schimmelfing, 1980). And the extent to which non-adherence dilutes or competes with potential health outcomes of exercise is still poorly defined. Shephard, Corey, & Kavanagh, (1981), for example, have shown that among post-myocardial infarction patients, exercise non-compliance was a critical prognosticator of both fatal and non-fatal recurrence, while other randomized clinical trials show no relationship between compliance and MI recurrence (Rechnitzer, Cunningham, Andrews, et al. 1983). Figures are not available regarding exercise compliance following prescription by a primary care provider, but data suggest that some individuals may be more likely to exercise outside a clinical setting (Wilhelmsen, Sanne, Elmfeldt, Grimby, Tibblim, & Wedel, 1975). The mental health outcomes for outpatients, however, may be less reliable for a home-conducted exercise program (Erdman & Duivenvoorden, 1983). The likelihood of starting and maintaining regular exercise outside a supervised setting is extremely difficult to estimate, but in one sample of dropouts from a cardiopulmonary rehabilitation exercise program (Bruce, Frederick, Bruce, & Fisher, 1976), 38% of the men and 40% of the women reported they continued a regular activity program on their own initiative. However, recent data indicate that approximately 50% of those who decide to enter a community exercise program report having experienced previous failures in adhering to such programs (Fitness Ontario, 1982; Martin, Dubbert, Katell, Thompson, Raczynski, Lake, Smith, Webster, Sikova, & Cohen, 1984).

THE EVIDENCE

It is useful to organize known correlates of programmatic exercise behavior into psychological, biological, and behavioral characteristics of the individual and into features of the exercise program or the setting where exercise occurs to include behavior modification techniques. This approach describes the types of variables that have been studied and may also serve a practical purpose since personal traits may assist in predicting the likelihood that a given individual will remain in an exercise program, while program features may be altered to accommodate the behavioral needs of participants. This approach is appealing since many of these factors are routinely assessed in pre-exercise diagnostic screening or they are part of the existing exercise program structure. These factors can usually be added with ease. A focus on stable characteristics also enhances the reliability of any relationships observed, and this can foster generalizability across studies. Unfortunately, it can also be argued that the predominant strategies used to study exercise adherence are self-limiting in promoting practical efficacy because they have not described exercise behavior as a process. Suggestions will be advanced throughout this chapter for encouraging a process approach that entertains the importance of interactions between the individual and the exercise setting, time stages during which different behavioral influences may predominate, and the possible influence of behavioral and psychological states on chronic behavior patterns (Dishman, 1982a).

BIOMEDICAL TRAITS AND LIFESTYLE HISTORY

Among post-myocardial infarction patients randomly assigned to rehabilitative exercise, of those initially screened as smokers holding blue collar occupations and involved in low intensity leisure activity, 80% eventually dropped out (Oldridge, 1979). This rate was increased to 95% among those who also were employed in occupations with low energy expenditure. However, this dropout profile applied to only about 15% of the total number of dropouts so its practical usefulness is restricted. Nevertheless, these results have been essentially stable within this population across various time periods ranging from three months to three years (Oldridge, et al., 1983). This enhances the generalizability of these findings to other rehabilitation settings. The presence of a cough or sputum was not a factor early on but emerged in later analyses (Oldridge, 1983). Likewise, at various times dropouts were likely to experience angina and to have had two or more MI's. Collectively, the patients with the highest risk for CHD, and those who might benefit the most from exercise, were most likely to drop out.

Our own work (Dishman, 1981a) has shown no relationship between MI and adherence, with a more heterogeneous group including apparently healthy, high risk, and documented CHD patients, while patients with low metabolic tolerance tended to adhere longer. Low metabolic tolerance was also related to severity of CHD symptoms. It was possible to classify those who dropped out in less than one month and those who adhered more than one-year using a symptomatic-asymptomatic dichotomy. This procedure's accuracy exceeded chance by 13%. Using body composition and metabolic tolerance, 44% of first month dropouts and 54% of those remaining after one year could be identified. Participants who were more disabled stayed with the program for a longer period of time (Dishman, 1981a).

Other studies show no relationship with metabolic tolerance (Dishman & Gettman, 1980; Franklin, 1984; Morgan, 1977; Ward & Morgan, 1984) or CHD symptomatology (Dishman & Gettman, 1980) while body weight or composition appear significant in some samples (Dishman, 1981b; Franklin, 1984; Massie & Shephard, 1971; Pollock, Foster, Salisbury, & Smith, 1982; Young & Ismail, 1977) but not in others (Bruce, et al., 1976; Morgan, 1977; Oldridge, et al., 1983; Ward & Morgan, 1984). Thus, biologic traits do not consistently show strong relationships with exercise behavior. For example, one study has shown dropouts possess lower left ventricular ejection fraction at rest and during peak exercise (Blumenthal, Williams, Wallace, Williams, & Needles, 1982), but this has not been seen in large studies of similar patient groups (e.g., Bruce, et. al., 1976).

I have proposed elsewhere (Dishman, 1981a), however, that biologic factors may influence behavior by interacting with psychological or setting factors to effect behavioral states that are reinforcing or aversive such as exercise sensations or chronic changes in disease symptomatology. This remains tenable but untested. However, data show that the common practice of relativizing exercise intensity to a standardized proportion of metabolic tolerance is ineffective in equating perceived discomfort during exercise (Ingjer & Dahl, 1979) and that low intensity activity may potentiate (Ballantyne, et al., 1978; Pollock, et al., 1977) but does not insure (Gwinup, 1975; Oldridge, et al., 1983) increased adherence.

Although studies imply that early program adherence (e.g., initial three months) predicts later adherence (e.g., 6 months and 12 months) (Dishman, 1982a), and recent data support this view (e.g., Frankel, Stevens, Dyer, & Craddick, 1983), little is known about the impact of previous physical activity outside the program setting. Several studies using self-report assessment of physical activity have shown no current day differences between former interscholastic and intercollegiate athletes and non-athletes (Dishman, 1981b; Morgan, 1981; Morgan, Montoye, Johnson, & Brown, 1983), whereas one early study has shown former athletes to become less active than former non-athletes by middle-age (Montoye, Van Huss, Olson, Pierson, & Hudec, 1957). Yet, it remains unclear if the exercise determinants are the same for the individual who begins habitual activity at middle-age compared with the person who has been active since childhood. Other studies support the findings of Oldridge and associate who found that inactive leisure time correlates with dropping out from a supervised exercise program (e.g., Franklin, 1984). However, our own data (Dishman, 1981b) revealed no correlation between program adherence and self-reported intensity, duration, or frequency of pre-enrollment exercise. This discrepancy may be specific to the population or activity, however, because a more recent study of a walking program for post menopausal women found differences in pre-program self-reports of daily stair climbing, number of city blocks walked per day, and daily caloric expenditure between adherents and dropouts (Bayles, Laporte, Petrini, Cauley, Slemenda, & Sandler, 1984).

These studies, together with those which consistently show blue collar workers and smokers to be more likely to drop out (Oldridge, et al., 1983), suggest that other behaviors from present day lifestyle may be good indicators of success in adhering to a regular exercise program. This is also consistent with results showing a high incidence of coronary prone behavior (Type A) among dropouts from cardiac rehabilitation at one month and one year

(Oldridge, 1977a; Oldridge, et al., 1978). Decisions to exercise may largely be influenced by previous lifestyle decisions or behaviors initially untied to exercise. It is likely that immediate day-to-day living can erode previous exercise habits or feelings held about exercise. This seems consistent with the inability of athletic history to predict programmatic exercise and the repeated observation that a spouse's attitude toward program involvement is apparently as great an influence on the participant's exercise behavior as his or her own attitude (Andrew, et al., 1981; Henizelmann & Bagley, 1970).

Other writers (e.g., Leventhal, Safer, Cleary, & Gutmann, 1980) have proposed reasons why life-style change can be important to exercise promotion. For example, a new or altered behavior is more likely to persist if it exists within a behavioral complex where specific acts facilitate or are compatible with each other and are cued by a range of environmental stimuli and reinforcements. The degree to which habitual exercise contributes to other risk behavior changes and the degree to which it is dependent on them has only recently been studied. For example, data from a successful stress management trial involving business executives who manifested a coronary prone behavior pattern (Roskies, Kearney, Spevak, Sunkis, Cohen, & Gilman, 1979) reported increased weekly recreational physical activity at six months followup even though they were instructed to maintain pre-experiment activity levels. Although reported diets did not change, subjects lost weight and had lower serum cholesterol; each change is consistent with increased exercise.

These data suggest that changes in other health behaviors may indirectly impact on exercise patterns. Moreover, a recent evaluation of a nine-month community fitness campaign. (Fitness Ontario, 1982) found that a generalized perception of lifestyle change was the single best estimate of self-reported activity levels, which were also related to reported changes in specific health behaviors of smoking, drinking, and weight control. In addition, when exercise and health behaviors are defined by observation, those who do not select an exercise program (Shephard, Morgan, Finucane, & Schimmelfing, 1980) and those who drop out (Oldridge, et al., 1978) have initially higher CHD risk profiles, and this is typical of multiple risk interventions (Meyers, et al., 1980). Also, epidemiologic evidence has shown an inverse relationship between smoking and habitual physical activity (Criqui, Wallace, Heiss, Mishkel, Schonfeld, & Jones, 1980) and smokers are less likely to enter (Shephard, et al., 1980) or remain in (Oldridge, et al., 1978; Massie & Shephard, 1971; Nye & Poulsen, 1974) a supervised exercise program.

These findings suggest a smoker is more likely to quit exercising than quit smoking (Taylor, Buskirk, & Remington, 1973) and reinforce the view that acquiring a healthy habit and breaking an unhealthy one are each difficult tasks. A similar picture emerges for weight control where exercise is known to facilitate a calorie deficit, but several studies show an inverse relationship between a heavy or fat body composition and exercise behavior (Brownell, Stunkard, &

Albaum, 1980; Dishman, 1981a; Dishman & Gettman, 1980; Gwinup, 1975; Young & Ismail, 1977; Massie & Shephard, 1971; Pollock, et al., 1982).

Although self-reports show perceived changes in health behavior are associated with exercise (Fitness Ontario, 1982; Gallup, 1984) existing objective data show little uniformity across health behaviors (Blair, Jacobs, & Powell, 1985). But, much remains to be learned in this area. It is not only critical in pragmatic terms of multiple risk factor reduction, but the validity of general models of health behavior change have yet to be demonstrated for physical activity.

PERSONALITY

Cross-sectional comparisons have shown habitually active adult males to be more extroverted than those who are sedentary (Lobstein, Mosbacher, & Ismail, 1983; Young & Ismail, 1977) but prospective studies have found extroverts to both be likely adherents (Blumenthal, Williams, Wallace, Williams, & Needle, 1982) and dropouts (Massie & Shephard, 1971). In a like manner, ego strength has been found to be positively related to program adherence among post-myocardial infarction patients (Blumenthal, et al., 1982) but unrelated to similar activity among college women (Dishman, Ickes, & Morgan, 1980).

Our work with a trait measure of self-motivation (Dishman, & Ickes, 1981) has been somewhat more consistent. Endurance athletes have consistently scored high on the scale (Freedson, Mihevic, Loutts, & Girondola, 1983; Knapp, Gutmann, Foster, & Pollock, 1984), and it has discriminated between adherents and dropouts across a wide variety of settings ranging from *athletic conditioning* (Dishman, Ickes, & Morgan, 1980; Knapp, et al., 1984), *adult fitness* (Dishman, 1983) *preventive medicine* (Dishman & Gettman, 1980), *cardiac rehabilitation* (Franklin, 1984) *commercial spas* (Olson & Zanna, 1982), *corporate fitness* (Stone, 1983), and *community based programs* (Martin, 1981). These programs have varied in length from five weeks to two years and have included men and women of various fitness levels. Other studies have shown no differences between adherents and dropouts on self-motivation in adult fitness (Gale, et al., 1984; Ward & Morgan, 1984), aerobic dance (Wankel, Yardley, & Graham, 1985); and interscholastic sport (Robinson & Carron, 1982). Even when mean score differences are small, the scale has been able to classify participants according to their exercise behavior with roughly 75% accuracy (Fitness Ontario, 1981; Olson, & Zanna, 1982; Stone, 1983). Our initial classification model (Dishman, Ickes, & Morgan, 1980) was 80% accurate when self-motivation scores were combined with body weight and composition, representing a 40% above chance estimate of behavior for dropouts and a 16% above chance rate for eventual adherents. This seems to support the usefulness of interactions between psychological and biological traits in accounting for exercise behavior.

Moreover, recent use of our original psychobiologic screening model by Ward & Morgan (1984) on a different sample represents the first attempt to actually predict prospective exercise behavior. These authors were able to predict *adherents* with 87% accuracy for males and 89% accuracy for females (a 40% gain above chance expectancy) but prediction of *dropouts* did not exceed chance. The prediction for adherents is encouraging from a practical standpoint since it represents the first true test of behavioral generalizability in the exercise adherence literature. However, the lack of specificity of the scale for dropouts is difficult to interpret and indicates the scale's usefulness may be restricted. This may mean that dropping out is psychometrically more complex than adhering or that our prediction model taps a dimension of self-selection rather than commitment as has been proposed elsewhere (Dishman & Ickes, 1981). Other data suggest that programs with strong social support or reinforcement may negate differences in self-motivation (Wankel, Yardley & Graham, 1985). The self-motivated individual may also be likely to leave a supervised program but continue a personal program.

An adherence role for motivational traits is conceptually consistent with a recently reported relationship between adherence and the Jenkins method of assessing Type A behavior (Rejeski, Morley, & Ribisl, 1984). Our unpublished data have shown a significant overlap between self-motivation and the Jenkins score; suggesting a common achievement motivation dimension (Dishman & Ickes, 1981).

PROGRAM FEATURES

Several studies suggest that programmatic features may have an impact on exercise behavior. These may interact with the predisposition or intention to be active and reduce or exacerbate existing psychological, behavioral, or lifestyle barriers to an exercise program. For example, logistic elements of perceived program inaccessibility or geographic inconvenience have been found to be related to the decision not to enter a program (Shephard, et al., 1980; Teraslinna, et al., 1969) and have been repeatedly related to dropout (Hanson, 1977, Andrew, et al., 1981; Gettman, Pollock, & Ward, 1983; Kavanagh, et al., 1973; Wilhelmsen, et al., 1975). This is consistent with anecdotal evidence of high attendance when alternative time schedules are made available (Franklin, 1984). Other experimental research (e.g., Thompson & Wankel, 1977) indicates that the *perception of choice* in selecting the activities to be employed is associated with increased attendance among female participants in a health club setting. Although perceived control over general health outcomes has not been related to exercise adherence (Dishman, Ickes, & Morgan, 1980), the importance of specific behavioral choices is well established in the self-regulation of other behaviors (e.g., Kirschenbaum, Tomarken, & Ordman, 1982). Moreover, these findings are conceptually similar to recent experimental evidence showing that flexible running distance goals set by participants according to daily preference were associated with higher attendance than inflexible goals established by an exercise leader (Martin, et al., 1984). Because failure to reach fitness goals has been reported as a correlate of dropping out (Danielson & Wanzel, 1977), flexible daily goals may help offset the "abstainer's fallacy" in which adherence to a behavior change is impeded by the belief that a temporary relapse inevitably leads to total relapse (Martin & Dubbert, 1984). This interpretation is consistent with our unpublished observations from both behavioral and psychometric measures (Dishman, 1981; 1983) that some individuals set excessively rigid and high goals compared to their biobehavioral skills and thus are doomed to failure at the outset. Additional experimental data have shown that chronic exercise behavior is enhanced when program structure is matched to personality factors related to the need for structure imposed by others or conversely the need for freedom of choice (Tu & Rothstein, 1979).

It has been clearly shown that excessive exercise volume can lead to program attrition due to injury (Pollock, et al., 1977). Among previously untrained males, (20 to 35 yrs.) running for twenty weeks at an intensity of 85 to 90% of maximum heart rate, a 17% dropout rate from injury can be expected to result when the daily duration is 45 minutes and the weekly frequency is three days. This may decrease to 6% at a duration of 30 minutes, five days per week because behaviorally significant injuries are unlikely with less duration and frequency at the same intensity. Thus, while excessive volume can directly contribute to drop out, it is less clear that intensity is the critical factor. Moreover, the typical preventive exercise program follows prescription guidelines for mode, intensity, duration, and frequency that create small risk for debilitating injury (American College of Sports Medicine, 1978). Other studies suggest that *perceived* exercise stress influences the decision to drop out. Even when exercise intensity has been relativized according to tolerance for vigorous physical activity, VO_2 max, participants who report subjectively greater discomfort are likely to discontinue (Ingjer & Dahl, 1979). Moreover, study has shown a lower dropout rate for a walking program in contrast to a more vigorous regime (Ballantyne, Clark, Dyker, Gillis, Henry, Hole, Muirdoch, Semple, & Stewart, 1978). However, in one sample of obese women only 32% completed an exercise program employing walking as the activity mode (Gwinup, 1975). It has also been reported that post-myocardial infarction patients may be more inclined to drop out of a low intensity recreational exercise program if they view it as offering little health benefit (Oldridge, et al., 1978). However, recent data from a three-year randomized trial of post MI patients have shown no differences in cumulative dropout rates (approximately 45%) between high volume exercise (less than 50% VO_2 max. predicted, two to six days per week) and low volume exercise (less than 50% VO_2 max. predicted, one day per week) (Oldridge, et al., 1983).

These findings collectively suggest that *preferred* exertion may be as important as perceived exertion in influencing exercise patterns, yet little is known about activity or intensity preferences. The energy demand of leisure time activities declines linearly with age (Montoye, 1975), but the origin of this change is not known. Among the middle-aged, however, participants who view exercise as having little health value select low intensity and low frequency activity (Sidney & Shephard, 1976). This suggests the importance of individual differences, but other studies show that during prolonged acute running (Farrell, Gates, Maksud, & Morgan, 1982) or bicycling (Morgan, 1983) the typical person will choose a work intensity that can be subjectively rated as either "moderately difficult" or "neither hard nor light", and this roughly corresponds to 60% to 80% of metabolic tolerance. This finding has been replicated in at least one study of chronic exercise (Morgan and Pollock, 1978) and suggests that program adherence may be enhanced if participants are permitted to initially select a preferred intensity. This remains to be tested, but there is presently little evidence to support the conventional wisdom that exercise intensity plays a major behavioral role in the typical preventive exercise program where the intensity prescription is relativized to 50% to 85% of a person's physiological tolerance for work.

This does not discount the significance of exercise sensations in interpreting the exercise experience, but it indicates that the specific role of bodily sensations in the adherence process remains unstudied. However, the observation that both acute running performance (Morgan, Horstman, Cymerman, & Stokes, 1983) and program adherence (Martin et al., 1984) have been facilitated by cognitive strategies designed to distract attention during exercise is consistent with a behavioral role for concrete exercise sensations. Moreover, it has long been accepted that music can increase voluntary metabolic effort and decrease perceived effort during exercise (Krestovnikoff, 1939), presumably by activation or distraction, and recent survey data show that many joggers prefer background music during running (Franklin, 1984).

BEHAVIOR MODIFICATION TECHNIQUES

One approach to facilitating exercise adherence is to identify program features or participant characteristics that appear to be behavioral barriers and then attempt to change them. Although this is theoretically a defensible strategy, it presents several pragmatic difficulties for implementation. Most known predictors of dropout from exercise programs are likely to be as difficult to change as is exercise behavior. Blue collar occupational status and the exercise attitudes of a spouse are not quickly altered, although spouse involvement has been used as a behavioral change agent (Brownell, Heckerman, Westlake, Hayes, & Monti, 1978; Sachs, 1982). Also, attempts to modify other behaviors related to a health promoting lifestyle, such as smoking and the coronary prone behavior pattern represent complex behavioral problems and the preferred modification strategies are not well understood. Likewise, changes in biologic factors such as body weight and composition, metabolic tolerance, and CHD risk or symptomatology depend to a significant degree on habitual exercise, the very behavior to which they may be inversely related. Programmatic factors such as geographic inconvenience are equally difficult to remedy, while exercise program directors are likely to resist modifying exercise volume or modality to meet the preferences of dropouts; desired fitness and health outcomes are largely activity-specific and dose dependent.

Although exercise prescriptions based on a juxtaposition of behavioral preference and biological need probably deserves close scrutiny in the future, a feasible alternative is to apply generalized principles and techniques of behavior modification in the hope they will effectively extend to health-related exercise settings. Reviews of the available technology for behavior management in exercise populations and its underlying principles can be found elsewhere (Epstein & Wing, 1980; Martin & Dubbert, 1984), and these can be broadly viewed as reinforcement and stimulus control techniques or as cognitive or self-regulation strategies.

Several studies have used written agreements, behavioral contracts and lotteries to increase exercise participation (Epstein, Wing, Thompson, & Griffin, 1980; Oldridge & Jones, 1983; Turner, Pooly & Sherman, 1976; Vance, 1976; Wysocki, Hall, Iwata, & Riordan, 1979). In these approaches, a person is required to sign an initial agreement to remain active for a certain period, and consequences of keeping or breaking the contract may be specified. The amount of exercise required can be determined by a random drawing. Other examples involved depositing money or valuable possessions that will be returned when the exercise program is successfully completed, or a behavioral contingency in which the attainment of a valued goal or activity is based upon first exercising for a predetermined amount (e.g., Allen & Iwata, 1980).

Various goal-setting and reinforcement techniques have also been effectively used. Most notable are those which employ self-monitoring (Oldridge & Jones, 1983), and stimulus control (Keefe & Blumenthal, 1980). In the former, participants are required to keep records of their completion of specific exercise behaviors, while the latter involves the use of objects, ideas, or other behaviors associated with exercise to create an environment that promotes exercise. While these approaches may capitalize on associational learning, they may also make it difficult to ignore a previous commitment to be active or a discrepancy between intention or commitment and actual behavior. When stimulus control techniques actually restructure the environment (e.g., taking a route home past a running park or keeping exercise clothes in the car or at the office) they may remove or diminish real (e.g., inconvenience) or imagined (e.g., excuses) barriers to activity.

Although it is not known how well behavior management principles compare with other possible programmatic changes (e.g., altering types of activity or intensity to fit behavioral or perceptual preference), studies applying behavioral techniques show a 60% to 80% adherence or attendance rate in many intervention studies compared to control rates of 40% to 60% (Martin & Dubbert, 1982; Martin, et al., 1984). These exceed the adherence rates found in the

typical exercise program where behavior interventions are not employed. However, they do not exceed those already observed (80% to 90%) in the most
successful existing clinical exercise programs (e.g., Kavanagh, et al., 1970,
1973, 1980; Greist, et al., 1979). This suggests that an alternative approach to
facilitating adherence might involve a component analysis of those programs
typically reporting high adherence rates and use of behavioral or program interventions to approximate or complement them. This has not been empirically
attempted in the exercise literature even though some authors have suggested
model programs based upon their clinical experiences (e.g., Franklin, 1984;
Oldridge, 1977; 1979b).

This alternative seems worthy of consideration because the typical research design used in behavior management interventions has not discounted
generalized treatment effects, therapist effects, or participant expectancy as
competing explanations to the presumably effective components of the intervention. Also, some of the most impressive intervention work completed (Martin,
et al., 1984) has relied heavily on a "treatment package" approach that encompasses a variety of behavior management principles (e.g., shaping, reinforcement control, stimulus control, behavioral contracting, cognitive strategies,
generalization, reinforcement fading and relapse inoculation). While these are
based on sound principles, and attempts have been made to make them compatible with program factors believed to influence adherence (e.g., convenience
and social support), their complexity does not allow specific evaluation of why
they work. Thus, these interventions have been unable to contribute much to
our understanding of why people do or do not adopt regular physical activity.

Moreover, the use of controlled placebo comparisons has been infrequent.
This is significant because in several instances where more than one intervention group has been used (e.g., Epstein, et al., 1980; King & Fredricksen,
1984; Martin, et al., 1984; Reid & Morgan, 1979; Stalonas, et al., 1978)
exercise behavior effects have often been similar for each treatment. Because it
has been reported that 50% of those who volunteer for behavior management
exercise programs claim to have previously attempted exercise on their own but
failed (Martin, et al., 1984), it is unclear to what degree these individuals may
be uniquely responsive to program packages that strongly emphasize social
support. In fact, it has been reported in one study that 53% of individuals who
have previously failed stated they had attempted exercise alone, even though
83% would have preferred to exercise with someone else (Martin, et al., 1980).
In a collective sense, behavior interventions have not discounted that a factor
common to the interaction between the client and treatment setting, notably
social reinforcement, principally accounts for the facilitation effects observed
(e.g., Stalonas, et al., 1978; Wankel, Yardley, & Graham, 1985).

In addition, most intervention studies have lasted for three to ten weeks
(e.g., Epstein, Wing, Koeske, Ossip & Beck, 1983, Wysocki, Hall, Iwata, &
Riordan, 1979; Allen & Iwata, 1980; Reid & Morgan, 1979; Epstein, Wing,
Thompson, & Griffin, 1980; Thompson & Wankel, 1980; Wankel & Thomp-

son, 1977; Wankel, Yardley, & Graham, 1985), while periods of three to twelve months or longer are of clinical significance to ongoing preventive medicine exercise programs. Thus, demonstration of a significant behavior change may not generalize to a programmatic advantage. Only about half of these intervention studies have examined followup recidivism after program termination, and few show maintenance of the intervention induced behavior change (Martin & Dubbert, 1982). Because, it has been suggested that a period of 10 to 20 weeks is necessary for psychological and biological training adaptations to occur that may provide reinforcing feedback (Greist, et al., 1979; American College of Sports Medicine, 1978), and that adherence through the initial three to six month period may enhance the likelihood of long term adherence (Dishman, 1982a) (Frankel, et al., 1983), short term behavior change packages may, however, offer pragmatic advantages even if they do not insure long term change. They might provide an important behavioral boost in the early stages of involvement that can be perpetuated by other programmatic factors or personal change that occurs later on. This seems borne out by recent studies where behavior change packages implemented within an ongoing program were effective for apparently healthy adults across a three-month period (Martin, et al., 1984) and for cardiac patients across a six-month period (Oldridge & Jones, 1983).

On the other hand, benefits are less clear for application of behavior modification procedures to increase exercise outside supervised programs. Several studies, for example, have demonstrated behavioral success using the Cooper aerobic point system as the dependent variable. (Kau & Fischer, 1974; Keefe & Blumenthal, 1980; Turner, Polly & Sherman, 1976; Wysocki, Hall, Iwata, & Riordan, 1979). However, clinical data on consecutive primary care patients who were prescribed exercise (Cantwell, Watt, & Piper, 1979) suggest that the volume of activity associated with both decreased CHD risk and high metabolic fitness, and which also approximates a weekly caloric expenditure of epidemiologic significance (e.g., Paffenbarger, Wing, & Hyde, 1978) corresponds to an aerobic point total two or more times greater than those achieved following behavior modification interventions.

MODELS OF EXERCISE BEHAVIOR

It has been proposed elsewhere (Dishman, 1982) that there remains a need to conceptualize models of exercise behavior that can lead to theoretical and applied research. This should particularly be beneficial due to the largely applied nature of the exercise adherence problem and the essentially descriptive nature of the relevant literature (Dishman, 1982b). The pragmatic search for technologies of behavioral prediction and control have yet to serve an applied advantage that is theoretically based and generalizable. The strongest predictive relationships have exceeded chance by only 13% to 40% (Dishman, 1981: Dishman & Gettman, 1980), and with one exception (Ward & Morgan, 1984) these have not been replicated in other samples. Also, the conditions under which exercise behavior can be explained or controlled have for the most part remained unspecified (Dishman, 1982b; Martin, et al., 1984), and it is not yet known who will benefit from behavior interventions.

ADHERENCE AS A PROCESS

While personal traits should be able to estimate the ability (e.g., fitness, health, body composition) and willingness (e.g., prior behavior, motivating or impeding symptoms) to adhere, just as program features should describe potential barriers (e.g., inconvenience of setting or time) or facilitators (e.g., effective leadership), the inherent limitations of a static descriptive model should be recognized. The lack of behavioral invariance across studies for personal traits and program factors may be largely due to transient interactions between the person and the exercise setting, and these may be best assessed as state measurements within the person, or trait changes, rather than static measures at program entry. Although at least two (Wankel, Yardley, & Graham, 1985) studies have shown program factors (e.g., rational decisions making and social support) can be effective motivators regardless of behavioral disposition at entry (i.e., self-motivation), I believe there is merit in examining models of exercise behavior within a dynamic interactive system analysis. This seems reinforced by the consensus that three critical components of effective behavior treatments (Leventhal & Cleary, 1979) are: 1) motivational factors (establishment of a goal, the decision and desire to change, and willingness to adapt to the process of change), 2) skills (knowing how to manage and change specific behaviors, and 3) a feedback process which systematically provides information and reinforcement regarding progress toward goals. Although some behavior modification approaches to exercise adherence have included parts of this process analysis (e.g., Martin, et al., 1984), most have not (Martin & Dubbert, 1982b), and an overview of the remaining exercise adherence literature quickly reveals the absence of a process orientation (Dishman, 1982a).

THE FALLACY OF SELF–EXPLANATION

One approach to measuring behavioral states simply asks participants why they dropped out. Among dropouts from a cardiopulmonary rehabilitation trial for 603 men and women, Bruce, et al., (1976) reported the following reasons: 1) *unavoidable,* i.e., due to schedule conflicts, excessive financial demands, moving (men, 34%; women 44%), 2) *medical* (men 21%; women 15%); 3) *unknown* (men 29%; women, 20%) and 4) *psychosocial* i.e., lack of interest and motivation, as well as personal conflicts involving families (men 16%; women 21%). Similarly, Oldridge (1979b) in a study of 592 post-myocardial infarction patients reported that among reasons for dropout, 20% were "unavoidable", 12% were medical, 5% were miscellaneous, and 63% were "psychosocial". While medical reasons and relocation are likely examples of true dropout factors which are easily corroborated, the explanatory limitations of other non-specific factors is apparent. Their reliability and generalizability is not known and they may actually reflect exercise motivation or perceptions of the program (i.e., "my schedule is too busy" may really indicate "I don't really want to exercise").

A similar, but more specific approach, was reported by Andrew & Parker, (1979) and Andrew, et al. (1981) and attempted to assess reactions to the exercise setting. Self-reports indicated program inaccessibility and schedule incompatibility with other commitments such as work were barriers to remaining active, as was lack of spouse support. Although these findings agree with other studies that have not relied on self-report (e.g., Hanson, 1977), their availability as stereotyped explanations or excuses (e.g., "I don't have time to exercise" or "my family needs me at home") (Fitness Ontario, 1981) must be discounted empirically before conclusions can be drawn about their true role in the adherence process (Dishman, 1982b). The need for psychometric approaches to self-report is illustrated by a recent study in which dropouts who reported the exercise facility was inconvenient actually lived closer than those who adhered (Gettman, Pollock, & Ward, 1983).

When actual characteristics of the exercise setting or participant traits are not used to interpret perceived reasons for dropping out, evaluation of their true behavioral meaning is not possible. Moreover, self-report approaches have typically not examined interactions among factors. For example, beliefs about the health benefits of exercise might be undermined by an unsupportive spouse, while the same inconveniences to which some participants attribute their decision to dropout can likely be overridden by the motivational traits and states of others. Although perceived reasons for exercise behavior and perceptions about attractive and aversive aspects of an exercise program (e.g., Andrew, et al., 1981) may be very real to an individual, reliance on self-views alone will not likely insure that changes made in corresponding program factors will lead to increased activity. Although changing the perceptions may offer a behavioral advantage (e.g., Thompson & Wankel, 1980), there is currently no standardized technology for assessing program perceptions (Dishman, 1982b).

Organizing existing data around a process model may eventually help explain why previous attempts to predict and control exercise behavior have not been more encouraging. For this purpose, behavioral traits and states related to: 1) the intention to exercise, 2) commitment to exercise, 3) getting the idea or being in a mood to exercise, and 4) reinforcement and dependence on exercise will be arbitrarily included. Available studies have, for the most part, examined these factors as traits, but they lend themselves to state measurement as well and in this respect may be particularly useful for predicting exercise at various stages throughout the adherence process (Dishman, 1982a). The observation that numerous traits can predict behavior early in a program, but not later, reinforces the validity of a process model for adherence (Dishman, 1982a; Oldridge, 1979b; Oldridge, et al., 1983; Ward & Morgan, 1984). These concepts have been chosen in the hope they can foster a multiple cause and interactive systems analysis rather than the pragmatic univariate description that has predominated past research. They may also provide a conceptual guide for defining target behaviors for behavioral interventions. In each instance this can add direction to the development of both theory and technologies for change.

INTENTION TO EXERCISE

Most studies have found little relationship between knowledge, beliefs and attitudes people hold about health behavior or exercise and actual adherence to an exercise program (Morgan, 1977; Dishman & Gettman, 1980; Andrew & Parker, 1979; Andrew, et al., 1981); although, those who expect health benefits have shown greater adherence in some studies (e.g., Andrew & Parker, 1979; Ho, et al., 1981). A similar state of affairs describes attempts to predict exercise behavior from measures of perceived physical competence (Dishman & Gettman, 1980; Morgan, 1977). This appears contrary to several social psychology models of general behavior (e.g., Ajzen & Fishbein, 1977), health behavior (e.g., Becker, 1974), and physical activity (Sonstroem, 1978).

Part of the inconsistency and confusion in exercise attitude research may, however, be explained by the absence of a valid technology for attitude assessment for specific populations (Safrit, Wood, & Dishman, 1985) or behaviors (Sonstroem, 1982). Other data suggest, however, that attitude measures may often assess attraction to activity or evaluative decisions about its worth but in the absence of an intention to be active, this will not likely lead to habitual activity (Sonstroem, 1982). This is supported by the observation that exercise attitudes can be related to the selection of activities (e.g., Sonstroem & Kamper; Sidney & Shephard, 1976; Harris, 1970), but not to continued involvement; an explanation is that regardless of actual behavior or the intention to be active, most people (including dropouts and adherents) both share a very favorable view about the health benefits of exercise (Andrew & Parker, 1979).

Survey data from several industrialized nations similar to the United States are consistent with the view that media campaigns which promote public involvement in recreational sport and exercise are very effective in enhancing knowledge and favorable attitudes (McIntosh, 1980). They appear equally ineffective in enhancing behavior, however, since estimated participation rates in these countries range from 10% to less than 50% (McIntosh, 1980). These figures are comparable to statistics observed recently in the United States (Harris, 1980) and Canada (Stephens, Jacob, & White, 1985). Reports from West Germany, Australia, and Canada indicate that only 10% to 17% of survey respondents who were aware of public promotions of physical activity acknowledged they were subsequently motivated to become more active (cf. Wankel, in press). Although these percentages are comparable to the impact of some programmatic behavior change strategies (e.g., Oldridge & Jones, 1983), they may exaggerate true behavior change and do not specify how many inactive individuals become active. Similar media based promotions in the United States have shown similar effects on knowledge about exercise, but no impact on actual physical activity levels (Meyer, Nash, McAlister, Maccoby, & Farquhar, 1980). The fact that other health risk behaviors have been more sensitive to media approaches (e.g., Meyer, et al., 1980) suggests that public motivation of exercise in the inactive may involve a largely unique process in comparison to other health behaviors.

Although cross sectional study has suggested that habitual exercisers have more formal education than inactive individuals (Harris, 1970; Yates, Leehey, & Shisslak, 1983), there is no convincing evidence that knowledge of the benefits of exercise corresponds with activity patterns. It may influence the intention to exercise, but this often does not translate into behavior (Fitness Ontario, 1981). A similar scene emerges for attitudes toward exercise and beliefs about health behavior. Neither have been shown to predict habitual exercise (Dishman & Gettman, 1980; Morgan, 1977) yet they may both be related to the intention to be active (Fitness Ontario, 1981), and this intention can be related to actual exercise behavior (Oldridge & Jones, 1983; Riddle, 1980; Sonstroem, 1982). Belief in the health benefits of exercise appears to consistently be a motivator of behavior only when there is evidence of a health deficiency or correctable disability (Andrew, et al., 1981; Dishman, 1982a).

Many clinical exercise programs continue to advocate a central role for an educational component (e.g., Franklin, 1984) even though the few available evaluations of this approach suggest it can be expected to have little lasting behavioral impact (e.g., Reid & Morgan, 1979). Recent theoretical views of exercise attitudes and knowledge (Olson & Zanna, 1981) suggest, however, that behaviorally specific attitude change strategies can be effective if they provide knowledge of specific behavioral goals, skills needed to implement a behavioral intention and if normative information (e.g., modeling or persuasion by a significant other) is included. Similar conclusions have been drawn for medical compliance in general (Haynes, Taylor, & Sackett, 1979) but remain to be tested.

Also, the results from several exercise studies can be interpreted within the framework of existing attitude and belief models even though the models themselves appear neither necessary nor sufficient to account for exercise behavior (Dishman, 1982d). For example, the health belief model (Becker, 1974) argues that compliance with a recommended health behavior is a function of: 1) perceived susceptibility to a particular disorder, 2) belief that negative outcomes will result from non-compliance, 3) an appraisal of potential benefits of the health behavior, 4) personal and environmental barriers to the behavior, and 5) internal (e.g., symptoms) or external (e.g., reminders) cues to action that make the advantages for the health behavior salient. In a previous attempt to conceptualize the available adherence literature (Dishman, 1982a), a considerable similarity with several of these components was observed, and they were quite useful in an organizational sense. Also, Oldridge (1979) has proposed that the health belief model be applied to the study of compliance in cardiac rehabilitation exercise programs. However, it is unclear if it has use for apparently healthy adults (Lindsay-Reid & Osborn, 1980), and it remains to be demonstrated that persuasion campaigns designed to facilitate an illness reducing behavior can operate effectively to promote initiation of healthy behaviors. Moreover, the health belief model has been shown to be behavior-specific (Haynes, Taylor, & Sackett, 1979).

COMMITMENT TO EXERCISE

Both behavioral and psychometric studies suggest that commitment is a measurable variable that relates to exercise adherence. Cross-sectional data show habitual runners to score high on a self-report measure of running commitment (Carmack & Martens, 1979; Thaxton, 1982), and this scale has also proven useful in predicting running behavior among college students enrolled in an endurance conditioning class (Dishman, 1983). Moreover, programs that require an initial fee to be deposited which is refunded only if all program sessions are completed (e.g., Gettman, Ward, & Hagan, 1982) frequently report higher than expected attendance rates, and this strategy has been successfully used as an exercise behavior modification method (Epstein, Wing, Thompson, & Griffin, 1980). Also, several studies show that contracts which specify a behavioral commitment are associated with increased adherence (Turner, Polly, & Sherman, 1976; Vance, 1976; Wysocki, et al., 1979). Oldridge & Jones (1983) recently reported a 65% compliance rate among cardiac rehabilitation exercise patients who signed an initial agreement to comply with the program for six months compared to a random control group rate of 42% and to a 20% compliance rate among exercisers who initially refused to sign the agreement.

Collectively, these findings indicate that both behavioral and self-report estimates of commitment to an exercise program obtained at the outset can be related to subsequent program adherence. Our work with the self-motivation scale (Dishman, Ickes, & Morgan, 1980; Dishman & Ickes, 1981) has represented one attempt to assess commitment at a psychometric level. Thus, while a technology is available to both measure and manipulate commitment, its origins and true role in adherence require further study. It is encouraging, though, that other attempts to assess commitment to behavior changes (e.g., quitting smoking) have also proven useful (e.g., Sjoberg & Johnson, 1978).

COGNITIONS, MOOD, AND EXERCISE BEHAVIOR

Despite the continued controversy in general psychology over the relative impact of thinking or feeling in the mediation of behavioral response (e.g., Lazarus, 1984; Zajonc, 1984), neither factor has been used as a model for directing research and practice in exercise behavior. There is, however, good reason to expect that each is important and that they may interact to influence a behavioral state at a given point in time. For example, at a self-regulatory level of behavior, several studies suggest that getting the idea to exercise can be an important influence on actual behavior much as ideations can be useful in other behavioral change attempts (e.g., Sjoberg & Samsonowitz, 1978). In a series of controlled intervention studies (Hoyt & Janis, 1975; Wankel & Thompson, 1977; Wankel, Yardley, & Graham, 1985), exercise behavior has been consistently enhanced following involvement in a rational decision-making procedure whereby an individual evaluates the costs and benefits anticipated from participation. Although the exact mechanism for this effect and its durability is not established, it is likely the act of evaluating serves as a reminder of a previous intention to exercise. This interpretation seems reinforced by the fact that this approach has been effective with dropouts and because other persuasion strategies were, by comparison, ineffective in facilitating reentry. A cognitive mechanism is also consistent with results from a field experiment (Brownell, Stunkard, & Albaum, 1980) that successfully used an exercise prompting sign placed in public transit settings to increase voluntary use of stairs rather than escalators. Similar exercise promoting effects have been seen for stimulus control approaches that take advantage of previous associations between exercise and ideas, objects, or routine behaviors (e.g., Keefe & Blumenthal, 1980).

Despite the well established link between mood and behavior, only recently have studies examined its role in exercise adherence. Descriptive data have been reported elsewhere showing a statistically significant elevation in psychometric depression among dropouts from a 32 week endurance training program for women's intercollegiate crew (Dishman, 1981) and it was suggested this might have signaled an overstress response to either training volume or life experiences which competed with remaining in the training program. Although speculative, this seemed consistent with the initially low self-motivation levels of the crew dropouts (Dishman, Ickes, & Morgan, 1980) and the demanding nature of the training regime. Recent training data from the U.S. Olympic speedskaters (Knapp, Guttman, Foster, & Pollock, 1984) have shown similar relationships in that athletes showing the least consistent training behavior also presented a chronic psychometric stress profile and were lower in self-motivation at the outset of training. Although these studies involved competitive athletes, the conditioning programs essentially differed only in volume of activity used in health-related exercise programs. Furthermore, at least four clinical studies confirm a relationship between habitual exercise patterns and mood-related variables. Lobstein, et al. (1983) found the MMPI depression scale to be the best discriminator between high fit active middle-aged men and those who were low fit and inactive. Blumenthal and associates (1982) have reported similar findings among a group of post myocardial infarction patients, observing dropouts to initially score higher on the MMPI depression scale, and this pattern agrees with data presented by Gentry (1980). Because these scales are believed to reflect relatively enduring characteristics, mood related factors may tap an energy or activation aspect of behavioral motivation or may indirectly signal chronic life conflicts that may create barriers to programmatic exercise. This speculation is further supported by a recent study (Ward & Morgan, 1984) showing adherents to initially present a more favorable composite mood profile than did dropouts, and this difference held at 10, 20, and 32 weeks of program involvement. Other cross-sectional data (Colt, et al., 1981) have implied exercise behavior may be motivated in some by management of symptoms in affective disorder.

It seems likely that day to day feeling states may directly relate to chronic exercise patterns since they may accumulate to form an aversive, or conversely attractive, disposition toward chronic activity. Also transient mood may reflect a state response of the exerciser to the demands of exercise or other life events that make daily exercise more or less likely (e.g., "I just don't feel like it today"). Moreover, since mood related personality traits have been shown to predict mood states even after a twenty year period (Morgan, Montoye, Johnson, & Brown, 1983) and because these have been related to lifestyle activity patterns, indicators of stable mood traits may predict a temperament that promotes activity.

EXERCISE REINFORCEMENT AND DEPENDENCE

The use of feedback has been cited as a unique component of exercise programs that report atypically high adherence and attendance rates (e.g., Kavanagh, Shephard, Chisholme, Qureshi, & Kennedy, 1980). Also, feedback is viewed as a fundamental aspect of both behavior change and learning (Leventhal & Cleary, 1980), and some attempts to facilitate exercise behavior have employed reinforcement strategies (Kau & Fischer, 1974; Keefe & Blumenthal, 1980; Martin, et al., 1984). Moreover, the undergirding significance of social reinforcement from the exercise setting and spouse support has been repeatedly implied by behavior change studies (Stalonas, et al., 1978) and exercise programs (Dishman, 1984; Oldridge, 1982). Finally, problems of motivation are typically cited by exercise clinicians when other reasons are not readily assignable, while several studies suggest that motivational traits may be among the most generalizable influence on exercise behavior (Dishman, 1984).

Despite this, virtually nothing is known of the process of reinforcement in exercise programs. A common wisdom suggests exercise should be enjoyable (Wankel, 1981), but the objective origins of enjoyment are not standardized for exercise participants or settings. Furthermore, while goal setting interventions have been used in an attempt to increase exercise adherence (Keefe & Blumenthal, 1980; Oldridge & Jones, 1983), no evidence describes the way in which self-motivated participants use goals to direct their exercise behavior (Dishman & Ickes, 1980). Also, the subjective meaning of exercise sensations as they change from aversive (e.g., discomfort) to reinforcing (e.g., signaling progress toward goals) has not been examined.

Because the study of exercise reinforcement appear central to understanding habitual exercise as a process, an exclusive preoccupation with dropping out (the predominant research strategy employed to this point) may be misplaced. Rather than viewing self-selection only as a bias that confounds the study of exercise influences and its effects (e.g., Oldridge & Jones, 1983), study of self-selection appears fundamental to determining who can benefit or adapt within programmatic exercise. This is supported because most known predictors of dropout are not sensitive to change, and exercise motivation has typically not been residualized from self-reported reasons for dropping out. How intractable are personal and lifestyle barriers to exercise among the inactive or dropout prone? Can we know what to change if we don't know why the active are active? The assumption that changing factors associated with inactivity will lead to activity has not been validated; describing the process of adhering may offer a complementary and equally pragmatic study alternative. Also, external validity for predicting adherence has received some support (e.g., Ward & Morgan, 1984), but the prediction of dropping out has not generalized across samples. Although asking the active why they exercise represents one study approach (e.g., Shephard, 1978, pp. 161–163), previous attempts have suffered from the same limitations described earlier for self-reports about dropping out. Other strategies may be preferred or complementary.

Aside from its abusive dimensions (Dishman, 1985; Morgan, 1979), there are reasons to believe the state of exercise dependence (Sachs, 1978) may provide one useful model of exercise reinforcement as a process. Psychometric, behavioral, and psychophysiological evidence (Baekeland, 1970; Hanson, Van Huss, & Strautneik, 1967; Thaxton, 1982) suggests that a state of exercise dependence exists and that it may describe an intrinsic motivational process which supports habitual exercise in a way inversely proportional to many of the situational barriers to exercise commonly perceived by the less active.

Dependence may actually integrate behavioral components such as intention, commitment, and exercise related cognitions and moods. If so, it can provide a common focus for exploring their interactions and can accommodate social, psychological, and biological sources of behavioral reinforcements. A dependence view of habitual exercise is also consistent with a stage analysis (Dishman, 1982a), whereby exercise may be reinforced by different factors as initial involvement progresses. In this sense, dependence on social reinforcement or self-control strategies during early adjustment to an exercise program may give way to later intrinsic reinforcements that can induce dependence. Although these might be biological (e.g., symptom abatement; Colt, et al., 1981; Greist, et al., 1979), or enhanced mood; (Morgan, 1985), there is no evidence that habitual exercise is associated with a biochemical dependence (Dishman, 1985; Morgan, 1985, Risch & Pickar, 1983). Behavioral dependence may, however, be related to self-identity (e.g., "I expect myself to exercise"), while clinical observations (Little, 1979; Yates, Leehey, & Shisslak, 1983) suggest preoccupation with exercise as a central definer of self may be both a fundamental intrinsic motivator and a precursor to exercise abuse when exaggerated.

A model of exercise dependence as a process is also consistent with the typical dropout pattern for programmatic exercise in which the attrition rate commonly plateaus after three or six months. Because biological changes with exercise training require a six to twenty week period (American College of Sports Medicine, 1978; Greist, et al., 1979; Morgan, Roberts, Brand, & Feinerman, 1970), many participants may require other reinforcements before the potential for intrinsic dependence can develop. However, the degree to which dependence may be acquired or is a predisposition remains untested, and this represents a major question over its usefulness as a pragmatic model of exercise reinforcement. Animal research (Hanson, et al., 1967) indicates that forced exercise during prepubescence can lead to increased spontaneous activity in adulthood. However, psychometric data from human adults (Morgan & Vogel, 1976) show that forced exercise can reduce attraction to physical activity. Moreover, clinical data suggest that abusive exercise dependence is largely related to premorbid vulnerability for crises of self-identity, (Dishman, 1985) suggesting that the degree to which exercise dependence develops is influenced by characteristics brought to the exercise setting by the individual. Furthermore, there are intriguing behavioral (Groos, 1898; Smith & Hagan, 1980), biological (Fagan, 1976), and biochemical (Redman & Armstrong, 1983) data to suggest that periodic physical activity is biologically motivated (Whalen & Simon, 1984); this may represent an innate behavioral rhythm that, for as yet unknown reasons, becomes disregulated across the human lifespan. Evidence from the exercise literature to discount this view could not be located.

PROBLEMS OF METHODOLOGY

There exists a need to standardize exercise programs, and the methods used for assessing exercise behavior and its correlates, if reproducible and generalizable results are to be obtained. The reported range in adherence rates of 13% in a cardiac rehabilitation program (Kentala, 1972) to 89% in a psychiatric sample (Greist, et al., 1979) attests to the magnitude of program diversity, and the absence of standardized psychometric and behavioral methods in studies examining psychological variables has been previously described.

Across samples, widely varying definitions of adherent or compliant behavior are used. For example, in two studies which observed cardiac rehabilitation patients across a 12 month period, one defined dropout as absence from supervised sessions for more than eight consecutive weeks (Oldridge, 1979b) while another (Dishman, 1981a) defined dropout as absence for 2 weeks. Although the most reliable influence on program adherence appears to be length of the program period studied, attempts have been made to contrast studies where the period of interest may range from less than one month (Dishman, 1981a) to 36 months (Oldridge, et al., 1983). The impact of this on results is best illustrated by the observation that some factors related to adherence early in a program can no longer be related later (e.g., Oldridge, 1979; Oldridge et al., 1983; Ward and Morgan, 1984).

There are also very different types and volumes of activity employed as the exercise stimulus for very different types of subjects. These have ranged from a study of male prison inmates who ran for twenty weeks at an intensity of 85 to 90% of maximum heart rate for a duration of 30 minutes, 5 days per week (Pollock, et al., 1977) to a group of urban females in a community based aerobic dance class that met for one and one-quarter hour once per week for ten weeks (Wankel, Yardley, & Graham, 1985). This diversity surely places varying behavioral demands on participants and provides differing social support systems, both of which can likely interact with characteristics of individuals to influence knowledge, attitudes, skills and motivation for exercise.

A need also exists to standardize the measure of exercise behavior (Laporte, Montoye, & Caspersen, 1985). This was reinforced by our own recent study (Dishman, 1983) of volitional self-paced running which showed different relationships between various measures of commitment depending on whether exercise behavior was viewed dichotomously as adherence vs. dropout, or as duration per session, sessions completed, or mileage. Measurement approaches have varied from retrospective self-report, to daily self-recording, to unobtrusive observation by program staff. Although several self-report tools for assessing occupational and leisure physical activity are available for population and group studies (Lindskog & Sivarajan, 1982; Paffenbarger, Wing, & Hyde, 1978; Reiff, Montoye, Remington, Napier, Metzner, & Epstein, 1967; Shapiro, Weinblatt, Frank, & Sayer, 1969; Taylor, Jacobs, Schucker, Knudsen, Leon, & Debacker, G., 1978; Yasin, S., Alderson, Marv, et al., 1967), they have not been employed in adherence studies which typically have used self-reports without concern for measurement error or actual validity. However, even validated questionnaires have been shown to have only a small overlap in their estimates of occupational activity (25%) and leisure time activity (16%) (Buskirk, Harris, Mendez, & Skinner, 1971), subsequently, their validity is not established. A newly developed 7-day recall interview shows promise for community-based activity assessment (Blair, Haskell, Ho, Paffenbarger, Vranizan, Farquhar, & Wood, 1985).

These results describe a serious problem for standardizing results for adherence studies that do not use direct observation of exercise and physical activity (Baranowski, Dworkin, Cieslik, Hooks, Clearman, Ray, Dunn, & Nader, 1984). Moreover, while questionnaires validated against biological estimates of activity (e.g., metabolic tolerance, body fat etc.) are useful in dichotomizing between high active and sedentary individuals, they are less accurate in distinguishing between levels of activity (Lindskog & Sivarajan, 1982; Taylor, et al., 1978). Most importantly perhaps, they also rely on recall and self-report, but their psychometric properties (i.e., reliability and behavioral validity) are largely unknown. For research purposes, continuous daily radiotelemetric monitoring of heart rate may be useful (Taylor, Kraemer, Bragg, Miles, Rule, Savis,

& Debusk, 1982), while a commercially available accelerometer that estimates caloric expenditure during exercise may offer an affordable and clinically useful alternative (Montoye, Washburn, Servais, Ertl, Webster, & Nagle, 1983). The usefulness of activity questionnaires from epidemiologic studies in detecting behaviorally significant amounts of activity variance remains unknown for small samples.

Whether objective estimates of exercise behavior indeed offer a clinically meaningful advantage over self-reported behavior remains to be tested, but at present it seems naive to accept unsupported claims about activity levels as valid and reliable. On the other hand, behavioral compliance does not insure that predicted biological change will occur (e.g., Haynes, et al., 1979; Rechnitzer, et al., 1983). Therefore, for practical and research purposes, it currently seems desirable to evaluate both subjective and objective evidence of exercise behavior when direct observation is not feasible.

There is also a need to determine a reliable baseline expectancy for exercise program compliance (i.e., by how much can exercise behavior be enhanced?). Clinical trials with post-myocardial infarction patients indicate that a substantial number of dropouts are due to medical contraindications. These have, for example, represented 14% to 21% (Bruce, et al., 1976), 22% (Oldridge, 1979), and 42% (Sanne, 1973; Wilhelmsen, Sanne, Elmfeldt et al., 1975) of dropouts from programs of 2, 3, and 4 years duration. Similarly, attrition due to injury has occurred in 17% of apparently healthy adult males randomly assigned to a 20 week running program of 45-minutes duration, 3 days per week at an intensity of 85 to 90% of maximum heart rate. Results such as these suggest that not only initial biomedical status, but also the volume of exercise employed in the exercise prescription, can contribute to an expected or baseline dropout rate that is not easily altered. There are other known nuisance factors, such as true conflicts in schedule and relocation, that cannot be controlled and should not be regarded as part of the exercise *behavior* problem.

A few studies report adherence rates as high as 89% at one-year (Greist, et al., 1979) and 77% to 81% at two-years (Kavanagh et al., 1973). But, these programs involved small groups (11 to 38 patients) and may represent a near maximum rate attainable under pragmatic restraints. This conclusion is also consistent with results from intervention studies using behavior management techniques; the most successful approaches have been associated with 10% to 20% increases above control expectancies and have not exceeded approximately 80% compliance (Martin & Dubbert, 1982; Martin, et al., 1984). Thus, the ultimate success of the pursuit toward increasing program compliance can only be evaluated against behavioral levels that are possible.

FUTURE CONCERNS

The thrust of research on habitual physical activity has focused on correlates of exercise behavior in supervised clinical or community programs. This pragmatic emphasis is understandable because non-compliance creates both a barrier to the delivery of services and a scientific confound in evaluating the efficacy of exercise training as a health or fitness intervention. It is also easier to measure exercise and its correlates in program settings. However, the lack of standardization of samples and methods in these studies raises important issues over the preferred allocation of resources for future research and application. Programmatic concerns over predicting and facilitating compliance with exercise prescription in clinical settings remain important, and a need still exists to better describe predictive interactions between characteristic traits and states of the participant and the exercise setting. This can be a particularly effective strategy within a given program when little change in the setting or the types of participants is anticipated. Prediction equations can be prospectively evaluated and refined, but this has not been done. Also, refinement of behavior management techniques toward exercise specificity, and isolation of their unique effects, provide a promising area for continued study and application. However, it can be argued that there may be advantages to viewing exercise behavior as a process, and previous attempts at conceptualizing existing findings were designed to foster more explanatory analyses for the future. In addition to highlighting this need, the limitations of an exclusively pragmatic perspective of exercise program adherence (i.e., based on segregated approaches to participant screening and program manipulation) also give reason to reexamine the endpoints to which the study of exercise behavior is directed.

Recent data from a community survey (Fitness Ontario, 1982) suggest that during a given sampling period (in this case nine months) one-half of those who are initially inactive, but intend to become active, will do so, while one-half of those initially active will become inactive. This is consistent with observations (Martin, et al., 1984) that one-half of individuals who self-select a supervised community exercise program report previous failures at remaining active. Because these figures roughly parallel dropout rates from the typical supervised exercise program, they illustrate a complex and as yet unaddressed dilemma for exercise promotion in public health. Namely, will health promotion through physical activity be best served through programmatic approaches to increase fitness or by community directed attempts to increase activity? Because each appear to have similar failure rates in changing behavior, (Ilmarinen & Fardy, 1977; Martin & Dubbert, 1982b) and both seem characterized by a strong self-selection bias, critical questions facing exercise and health science may include decisions about who is most likely to benefit from which approach rather than the comparative advantage of one over the other. Clinical trials bear this out. For example, one study of obese adolescents (Epstein, Wing, Koeske, Ossip, & Beck, 1983) has found similar short term weight loss between conditions of programmatic exercise and increased routine physical activity, but the routine activity group maintained the effect for a longer period during followup. This suggests that the method of choice for physical activity intervention may depend upon the desired outcome and may be more behaviorally and biologically complex than previously acknowledged. Although cross-sectional data from both adult males (Cooper, Pollock, Martin, White, Linnerud, & Jackson, 1976) and females (Gibbons, Blair, Cooper, & Smith, 1983) show an inverse relationship between metabolic fitness and coronary heart disease risk factors, and experimental data convincingly show that exercise training increases metabolic fitness (American College of Sports Medicine, 1978), while regulating plasma lipoproteins (Wood, Haskell, Blair, Williams, Krauss, Lindgren, Albers, Ho, & Farquhar, 1983), explanations underlying its correlational link with cardiovascular health remain obscure (Haskell, 1979). Moreover, a recent randomized clinical exercise trial with post-myocardial infarction patients showed no difference in recurrence rates between high intensity and low intensity exercise groups even though fitness gains were commensurate with intensity (Rechnitzer, et al., 1983). Both groups showed a 45% dropout rate across the 3 year study period, but this was not related to recurrence.

    Thus, while epidemiologic studies continue to show inverse relationships between a physically active lifestyle and both morbidity and mortality for coronary heart disease (Blair, 1982), it remains to be determined for whom implementation of programmatic exercise is an effective or preferred health intervention from either behavioral or health and disease perspectives. A similar scene exists for other dimensions of the exercise and health relationship. Both, cross-sectional and quasi-experimental studies show a consistent association between exercise programs, fitness, and mental health (Dishman, 1985; Morgan, 1979), yet randomized clinical trials show conflicting results (e.g., Greist, et al., 1979; Morgan & Pollock, 1978; Stern & Cleary, 1982).

    These findings suggest, both from standpoints of an epidemiologic rationale for exercise promotion and the possibly intractable self-selection barrier to supervised exercise training for many individuals, that alternatives to the traditional fitness approach to exercise as a healthy behavior warrant exploration. Field studies show the feasibility of increasing energy expenditure through increased routine daily physical activity (e.g., Brownell, et al., 1980; Epstein, et al., 1983), and a lifestyle characterized by moderately intense routine activity is known to retard the decline in metabolic fitness typically seen with age (Epstein, Keren, Udassin, & Shapriro, 1981). Moreover, recent field research (Berger & Owen, 1983) also suggests positive psychological outcomes can be associated with routine physical activity, even though research on programmatic exercise suggests that the relationship between exercise and enhanced mood is dose dependent (Morgan, 1979). The feasibility of altering popular recreation patterns to a health and fitness advantage, or using them as behavioral models for increased programmatic adherence, remains largely unexplored (Wankel, 1981). It is important to note, however, that a "lifestyle" focus on increasing habitual physical activity will likely prove equally problematic in a behavioral sense, because it is well established that preferred leisure time activity declines steadily with age (Montoye, 1975) and because inactive leisure time has been shown to be related to dropping out from exercise programs among some people (Oldridge, et al., 1983).

In unison, available evidence reveals that behavioral problems associated with programmed exercise and with routine or leisure activity seem equally complex and intertwined, and this complexity reveals a fundamental flaw in previous strategies used in exercise adherence. That is, the three major service agencies currently examining exercise as a healthy behavior (what Leventhal & Cleary, (1979) refer to as 1) sociocultural e.g., public health promotion campaigns; 2) self-regulatory, e.g., behavior management and personal skill development; and 3) health care providers, e.g., adherence or compliance to supervised prescription seem to have operated largely without the knowledge or counsel of others. This has perpetuated application of three essentially distinct technologies at the expense of developing theoretical models of exercise behavior, and this has undoubtedly limited the practical impact of each approach. Investigative strategies have appeared technology-bound in the questions asked, the methods used, and their potential impact. *Clinical exercise programs* have examined factors most easily assessed within existing biomedical screening protocols, have relied on self-report taken at single time periods without concern for psychometric and kinematic issues of measurement error and validity, or have altered program features on the basis of intuition or ease rather than evidence; psychological methods of inquiry have been essentially ignored (Oldridge, 1982). *Behavioral interventions* have for the most part applied change techniques based on generalized principles without regard for biological needs or behavioral deficits that may be unique to the exerciser or the exercise setting or for behavioral endpoints that are compatible with the health and fitness objectives of programmatic exercise. Finally, *public health promotions* (e.g., media campaigns) have largely focused on the very factors shown by-and-large to be unrelated to both programmatic and leisure exercise behavior, namely knowledge and attitude.

From a pragmatic standpoint, this segregation is, of course, understandable because each approach is limited by training and the technology available to it. From the standpoint of theoretical and applied utility, however, it becomes clear that future efforts from exercise science, behavioral medicine, and public health, must become better integrated. This seems reinforced by three questions common to each domain that remain unanswered. Namely, 1) Who most benefits from exercise programs and who may better respond to "lifestyle" changes in physical activity (i.e., hard paths vs. soft paths to behavioral health)? 2) Can we motivate those who will benefit but are not motivated to be active? 3) What are the preferred ways to support or teach those who are motivated to change, but cannot?

6

EXERCISE AND MEDICATION IN THE PSYCHIATRIC PATIENT

Egil W. Martinsen

INTRODUCTION

Until the last two decades, most physicians have paid little attention to the life styles adopted by their patients. For many years, the most common advice to patients was to take it easy, and rest was considered the best way of preserving good health. Research has shown that there is an interaction between life style and illness. Studies indicate that exercise can be an effective tool in the prevention and treatment of various diseases, and this is especially true for somatic diseases. Perhaps the best example is the use of exercise in rehabilitation of patients after a cardiac infarction. A great number of these patients are receiving pharmacological agents for their disease, with the most important group of drugs being the beta blockers. Furthermore, there is a growing number of research reports concerning the interaction between the use of beta blockers and exercise. These investigations, along with clinical experience, have shown that exercise is not contraindicated for patients receiving beta blocking agents.

There was a pharmacological revolution in psychiatry during the 1950's with the introduction of the phenothiazines in the treatment of psychoses and the tricyclic antidepressants in the treatment of depressions, and a high percentage of psychiatric patients currently receive these and other psychotropic drugs. These two classes of drugs have a wide range of somatic side effects, and the most important are the effects on the cardiovascular system. Like other health professionals, psychiatrists have paid little attention to their patients' passive, sedate life styles. In recent years, however, research has shown that psychiatric patients generally are in poor physical condition, and there is some evidence that regular exercise may lead to improved mental health (Morgan, 1984).

Since many psychiatric patients are receiving psychotropic drugs, the question arises: To what extent does the use of medication interact with the effects of exercise. Unlike the situation in cardiology and physical rehabilitation medicine, little interest has been paid to this issue by psychiatrists, and very little research exists on this topic. The importance and necessity of systematic research on this question becomes readily apparent when one considers the increasing popularity of exercise therapy (Morgan, 1985) in concert with the widespread usage of psychotropic drugs in the treatment of psychiatric patients.

The purpose of this discussion will be to focus on selected problems of a central nature in this area. The limited research involving the influence of exercise on patients receiving the most important groups of psychotropic drugs (i.e., the major tranquillizers, the tricyclic antidepressants, lithium and the minor tranquillizers) will be reviewed. The interaction between beta blocking agents and exercise will also be discussed. This happens to be a very commonly used group of drugs; many psychiatric patients receive these drugs for somatic disorders; and they seem to have effects on mental stress response as well (Jefferson, 1974). A controlled study performed at the Modum Bads Nerve-sanatorium will be described, and this research dealt with the effects of aerobic exercise on hospitalized, depressed patients. Finally, a review of case material involving the influence of exercise on patients receiving specific drug treatment at the time of exercise intervention will be presented.

RELEVANT PROBLEMS

Many important questions arise when one attempts to focus on the interaction between exercise and medication. The following questions represent some of the more important topics in this area.

1. What is the effects of medication on the cardiovascular response to exercise? Can medication lead to impairment of cardiac function as reflected by a decrease in work capacity and failure of blood pressure to rise normally during exercise? Can medication attenuate the effect of exercise programs, and affect the motivation for exercise?
2. Is there a risk of special complications to exercise during pharmacological treatment?
3. Can exercise reduce or increase the side effects of medication?
4. Can exercise increase or reduce the therapeutic effect of medication?
5. Can exercise replace medication?

LITERATURE REVIEW

This section will focus on the most important psychopharmacological agents and the beta blockers. An effort will be made to answer some of the questions raised in the previous section.

Neuroleptics

The neuroleptics have a wide range of effects on the body, and some of these interfere with the capacity and motivation to exercise. Drowsiness is a frequent complaint with the high-dose phenothiazines. The effect is most pronounced initially, and will often be markedly reduced after the first 2–3 weeks of treatment. Parkinsonism is another common side effect, which reduces the capacity and ability for exercise. Weight increase will, of course, reduce physical capacity, but exercise should theoretically be an effective way to deal with this side effect.

Neuroleptics, especially the high-dose compounds, have an adrenolytic and a less pronounced anticholinergic effect, which will affect the cardiovascular system and its response to exercise. Orthostatic hypotension is often seen initially in the treatment with phenothiazines, and is particularly characteristic of treatment with the high-dose compounds. This effect will often subside or disappear after some time of treatment. Tachycardia will often accompany the hypotension, but may also appear as an isolated phenomenon. The phenothiazines have a quinidine-like effect on the electrocardiogram (ECG), but these changes rarely have clinical importance.

Long term treatment with chlorpromazine results in reduction of the mean arterial blood pressure in the upright position (Korol, Land, & Brown, 1965). Carlsson, Dencker, Grimby and Häggendal (1968a) have performed several studies on the physiological effects of medication on patients receiving large doses of chlorpromazine (1.5–3.6 g/day). They found that large doses of chlorpromazine tend to reduce the stroke volume, leading to a reduction of cardiac output and arterial blood pressuring during exercise. Carlsson, Dencker, Grimby, and Häggendal (1967) also reported that the concentration of noradrenaline in blood plasma and urine is increased with chlorpromazine treatment. This difference is present at rest, and it is still more striking during exercise (Carlsson, et al., 1967). The normal physiological response to regular exercise programs is altered by chlorpromazine use. According to Carlsson, Dencker, Grimby, and Häggendal (1968b), the reduction of heart rate and blood lactate at a given work load is less consistent with patients treated with chlorpromazine. The high level of noradrenaline during exercise is reduced, however, after a period of aerobic training (Carlsson et al., 1968b).

The small stroke volume and the fall in arterial blood pressuring during exercise are factors that limit physical work performance. Some cases of sudden death among patients receiving phenothiazines may have been due partly to this maladaption of circulation. Another possible explanation may be the large increase in the blood level of noradrenaline during physical activity among physically inactive patients receiving phenothiazines.

It may be difficult for patients to exercise while receiving phenothiazines, because of the side effects of drowsiness, orthostatic hypotension and Parkinsonism. Nevertheless, exercise is indicated for these patients, both to increase their physical work capacity, and to reduce the level of noradrenaline in blood plasma.

At this time, it is not possible to draw any conclusions regarding the effect of fitness training on *psychotic* symptomatology (Folkins & Sime, 1981). However, these drugs are also used as tranquillizers for *neurotic* disturbances, and it is possible that regular exercise might give a tranquillizing effect comparable to that of these drugs. This hypothesis remains to be tested, and it is important to realize that studies addressing the effects of smaller doses of chlorpromazine and of other neuroleptics on exercise performance, do not exist at this time.

Tricyclic Antidepressants

The structure of tricyclic antidepressant drugs is similar to that of the phenothiazine group of the major tranquillizers (e.g., chlorpromzine), and their pharmacological actions are both anticholinergic and adrenolytic. These drugs have different adverse effects on the cardiovascular system. A common side effect of the tricyclic antidepressants is increased heart rate, which is probably related to their anticholinergic effect on the vagus. Glassman and Bigger (1981) suggested that the only significant adverse cardiovascular effect of tricyclic antidepressants is healthy adults taking therapeutic doses, is orthostatic hypotension. A decrease in blood pressure noted with tricyclic antidepressants is probably related to their noradrenergic blocking effect (Jefferson, 1975). Veith, Raskin and Coldwell (1981) found no change in left ventricular function in cardiac patients taking either doxepin or imipramine. There is little evidence that tricyclic antidepressants at therapeutic doses, reduce the mechanical function of the heart (Glassman & Bigger, 1981).

Some studies show that therapeutic doses of tricyclic antidepressants affect cardiac conduction, producing a significant prolongation of the QRS and PR intervals of the ECG (Vohra, Burrows & Sloma, 1975). Veith et al., (1982), however, failed to observe such an effect. The tricyclic antidepressants are known to resemble quinidine with respect to their effect on cardiac rhythm (Glassman & Bigger, 1981). At therapeutic doses, both imipramine and doxepin have been reported to reverse some arythmias. At high doses, or overdoses, tricyclic antidepressants produce arythmias (Luchins, 1983). As for the phenothiazines, drowsiness and fatigue are common complaints, especially at the start of the treatment, and this will reduce the motivation and ability for exercise. Another problem with these drugs is the associated increase in body weight. Studies of the effect of these drugs during submaximal or maximal exercise have not been performed (Powles, 1981).

There have been attempts to explain the antidepressive effect of exercise on the basis of the same mechanism thought to operate with the tricyclic antidepressants, electroconvulsive therapy (ECT), and sleep deprivation. These explanations are usually based upon the monoamine hypothesis (Morgan, 1985).

The reasons for this are that exercise seems to have an antidepressive effect, and the effects of exercise on sleep disturbances resemble those of other treatment methods for depressions (Ransford, 1982). According to this view, one could speculate that exercise would potentiate the effects of tricyclic antidepressants and vice versa. On the other hand, tricyclic antidepressants seem to have their best effects on the more severe depressions, whereas the antidepressive effect of exercise is best documented in patients suffering from moderate to mild depressions. Furthermore, patients with mild depressions often do not respond well to antidepressant medication. Studies comparing the antidepressive effect of exercise and tricyclic antidepressants on different types of depressions, and studies trying to investigate whether exercise and medication can potentiate each other, do not exist.

Several studies indicate that imipramine treatment leads to a reduction of anxiety, both phobic and free floating type (Zitrin, Klein, & Woerner, 1978). The same authors, however, report a high frequency of medication side effects. About 20% of these patients were exquisitely sensitive to imipramine and responded to the initial 25 mg dose with insomnia, jitterness, irritability and unusual energy (Zitrin et al., 1980). A great number of these patients have been treated at Modum Bads Nervesanatorium with the same effect. These patients, in particular, seem to react negatively on the amphetamine-like, activating effect of imipramine. These side effects might well be determined in part by the patient's personality profile, i.e., their fear of self assertiveness, of losing attachment and so on (Holm, 1984). A logical question becomes: Will these patients have less unpleasant side effects when the psychiatric treatment is combined with exercise? Exercise might, for example, reduce the subjective feelings of side effects by channeling the released extra energy in a manner acceptable for the patients.

Lithium

Lithium is used extensively in the treatment of depression, but its effects on exercise performance in the human are unknown (Powles, 1981). It is known, however, that lithium causes reversible T-wave changes in the ECG and reduces myocardial contractility in dogs (Singer & Rotenberg, 1973).

Minor Tranquillizers

The minor tranquillizers have less extensive effects on the cardiovascular system. A few studies have addressed the cardiovascular effects of these drugs. In resting dogs, intravenous diazepam and chlordiazepoxide produce an increase in coronary blood flow and cardiac output, and a decrease in myocardial contractile forces, arterial blood pressure and heart rate (Daniell, 1975). In resting humans, diazepam increases coronary blood flow in normals, and even more so in patients with coronary disease (Gooch, Natarajan, & Goldberg, 1974). The effect of these drugs in humans performing upright exercise is unknown (Powles, 1981).

Several studies indicate that regular exercise leads to a reduction in anxiety, muscular tension and sleep disturbances. An important question is related to whether or not exercise can replace minor tranquillizers. deVries and Adams (1972) compared the tranquillizing effect of single doses of exercise and meprobamate (400 mg) with respect to reduction of muscular action potential level and heart rate. These investigators reported that exercise had a significantly greater effect upon the resting muscle action potential than did meprobamate. This led to the conclusion that exercise must not be overlooked when a tranquillizer effect is desired. Can exercise really replace drugs in the treatment of disturbances of this nature? The widespread use of these drugs, the risk of abuse, drug dependence and other side effects certainly makes this an important area for further studies.

Beta-adrenergic Blocking Agents

The use of beta-adrenergic blocking agents is now widely established in the management of a variety of conditions, such as angina pectoris, hypertension, obstructive cardiomyopathy and migraine. The possible protective effect after myocardial infarction has further increased their use. Some authors claim that beta blockers are also effective in the treatment of emotional disturbances, such as anxiety (Michael, 1980). Beta-adrenergic blocking agents might, in theory, affect exercise capacity by several distinct mechanisms. First, they depress the total cardiac output by reduction of the heart rate through antagonism of cardiac $beta_1$-adrenoreceptors. Second, they impair the blood supply to the muscles by blocking the $beta_2$-adrenoreceptors in the walls of the blood vessels. Third, they affect the metabolism of fatty acids and glucose, and they might have a direct effect on muscular contraction (Breckenridge, 1982).

Although different research reports give somewhat conflicting results, it now seems generally accepted that beta-adrenergic blocking agents impair a person's exercise performance, and both endurance time and maximal oxygen uptake are reduced (Andersen, Bye, Perry, Hamor, Theobald, & Nyberg, 1979). The size of the reduction will vary from person to person and depends on the dosage of the drug given. A reduction in cardiac output up to 22% in normal subjects at maximal work has been reported (Epstein, Robinson, Kahler, & Braunwald, 1965). Another important question is the following: What is the effect of chronic beta-adrenergic blockade on the ability to obtain a cardiovascular training effect from an exercise conditioning program? The studies addressing this topic give conflicting results. One study has shown that aerobic exercise provides no increase in aerobic capacity in patients with coronary artery disease who are receiving beta-blockers (Malmborg, Isaccson, & Kalli Vroussis, 1974). Another study showed that the use of beta-blockers markedly attenuated the cardiovascular conditioning effects of exercise in normal subjects, and the authors suggested that beta-adrenergic stimulation is essential in exercise conditioning (Sable, Brammell, Sheehan, Nies, Gerber, & Horwitz, 1982). There are at least four other studies on patients with coronary heart disease showing that substantial training effects can be achieved despite the use of therapeutic doses of beta blockers (Vanhees, Fagard, & Amery, 1982). This is important since the training heart rates are consistently reduced in patients receiving therapeutic doses of beta blocking agents. While there are diverging views, most experts today seem to think that training effects may be achieved while using beta blockers.

A sensation of muscle fatigue while exercising is a common problem in patients using beta blockers. The reason for this discomfort is not clear. One possibility is the decreased blood flow to the exercising muscles by blocking of the beta-adrenoreceptors in the walls of the blood vessels. Metabolic changes with reduced substrate supply to the muscles is another: The blood level of glucose and free fatty acids fall during exercise while using beta blockers (Lundborg, Åström, Bengtsson, Fellenius, von Schenck, Svensson, & Smith, 1981). One study showed that beta blockade influenced serum potassium levels during and after exercise (Carlsson, Fellenius, Lundberg, & Svensson, 1978), and there may be an effect directly on the muscles. Theoretically, beta blockers by virtue of their membrane-stabilizing action may effect neuromuscular activity at the motor end place, and this may contribute to muscular fatigue (Bowman, 1980). Hypoglycemia induced by exercise is another problem (Uusitupa, Aro, & Pietkainen, 1980). The normal response of blood glucose to exercise as well as to hypoglycemic is reduced by beta blockers, presumably by inhibition of the $beta_2$-adrenoreceptor mediated liver glycogenolysis (Bewsher, 1967). The reduction of warmth production by reduced lipolysis and reduced trembling may be of importance for maximal exercise especially in cold climates (Aksnes, 1977).

An important applied question deals with the kinds of beta blockers that are most comfortable for runners. Theoretically, $beta_1$-selective blockers might be expected to have an advantage, but this has been hard to prove in scientific research studies. An alternation in dose or a change of the particular agent may be beneficial in treating patients who report symptoms of undue fatigue and compromised exercise performance. Beta blockers will have to be chosen on the basis of trial and error at present for patients receiving exercise prescriptions.

The use of beta blockers reduces the capacity to perform exercise. Opinions differ as to whether or not the normal training effect is attenuated by using these drugs. Common complaints are exercise-induced muscular fatigue and hypoglycemia, and patients performing endurance exercise while on beta blockers are advised to ingest suitable substrates for the muscles to prevent symptom-producing hypoglycemia.

Hospitalized psychiatric patients often receive psychopharmacological agents as part of their therapy, and many receive beta blockers as well. Exercise is a relatively new therapeutic approach. A controlled study will be reviewed in the next section. The purpose of the study was to assess the antidepressive effect of exercise on hospitalized, depressed patients.

THE EFFECT OF EXERCISE ON DEPRESSION: REVIEW OF A CONTROLLED STUDY

This investigation involved 49 hospitalized male and female patients who ranged in age from 17–60 years (mean = 40). The patients satisfied the DSM-III criteria for Major depression: Single Episode (296.2 × = 2.3) and Recurrent (296.3 × = 2.3). Psychotic patients and those with somatic contraindications for exercise were excluded. The mean number of years since the first depressive episode was 11 (range 0–35), and the mean number of previous episodes was 8 (range 0–50). The duration of the present episode was more than 6 months for 33 patients. All the patients were on individual psychotherapy and occupation therapy, and 23 patients received tricyclic antidepressants (Martinsen, Medhus, & Sandvik, 1985).

The patients were randomly assigned to exercise and control groups. The exercise group underwent a 9 week training program. The training included walking, jogging, bicycling, skiing and swimming at 50–70 percent of predicted maximal aerobic capacity, and the exercise was performed for one hour, three times per week. The control group attended ordinary occupational therapy while the training group was exercising. The overall treatment program was kept as similar as possible for the two groups with the exception of the exercise intervention.

The effect variables were registered at inclusion and after 3, 6, and 9 weeks of treatment. The dependent variable was depression as measured by the Beck Depression Inventory, and the depression subscale of the Comprehensive Psychopathological Rating Scale (CPRS) (Åsberg, Perris, Schalling, & Sedvall, 1978). Physical condition was assessed with a submaximal bicycle ergometer test designed to predict maximum oxygen uptake (Åstrand & Rodal, 1977).

Four patients in the training group dropped out of the study. Two of the drop-outs discontinued due to mild sport injuries, one to lack of training motivation, and one was discharged. Two patients in the control group were discharged during the course of the study. Discharges were not under the control of the project leaders. Twenty-four patients from the exercise group completed the study, combined with 19 in the control group. Fourteen patients in the control group and 9 patients in the training group also received tricyclic antidepressant medication in doses varying from 50–150 mg/d. Seven patients in the training group had mild sport injuries which healed within a few weeks, and there were no serious complications to the exercise. For the efficacy variables, the evaluation of p-values was based on differences from inclusion to after 9 weeks of treatment.

There was a high correlation between the CPRS and Beck depression scores (r = 0.70). The mean reduction in the CPRS and Beck scores were significantly larger (P < 0.05) in the training group than in the control group. The antidepressive effect seemed better for males than for females. Mean maximum uptake increased more in the training group than in the control group (P < 0.001) as expected.

For all the items in the CPRS-scale, the observed mean reductions were largest in the training group. The difference in favor of aerobic exercise was largest on the items: inner tension, depressive thinking, concentration difficulties, sleep disturbances and observed muscular tension. In the training group, the correlation between the increase in maximum oxygen uptake and the reduction in CPRS score was higher for males (r = 0.40) than for females (r = —0.13).

The study by Martinsen et al., (1985) shows that it is possible to carry out physical training programs for hospitalized, depressed patients up to 60 years old, with positive effects on their physical condition. Aerobic exercise has an antidepressant effect on these patients, and this corresponds with the findings in other investigations with physical training for young and mildly depressed patients (Greist, Klein, Eischens, Faris, Gurman, & Morgan, 1979).

The antidepressive effect of the training program was greater for males than for females. An opposite trend was reported by Folkins, Lynch and Gardner (1972). Possible explanations for this discrepancy may be: (1) different effects of exercise on different types of depression, (2) differences in the training programs, and/or (3) chance. In the present study, a positive correlation was found between the antidepressive effect and the increase in physical condition for males. This relationship has not been reported in previous studies.

Several hypotheses have been postulated in an attempt to explain the psychological effect of exercise, and both biological and psychological explanations have been offered. One of the latest hypotheses was advanced by Bahrke and Morgan (1978), and it addressed the issue of whether exercise per se is the crucial variable in reduction of anxiety. Their work suggests that comparable anti-anxiety effects can be produced with simple rest or distraction. The present study indicates that a strong positive correlation exists between the intensity of exercise and the antidepressive effect for males. This finding suggests that the effect of exercise is more than mere distraction, and aerobic exercise seems to have a genuine antidepressive effect. The present work involved a long term training stimulus (e.g., 9 weeks), whereas the report by Bahrke and Morgan (1978) was based upon acute exercise. The present findings need to be replicated in new experiments and with new groups of patients. Many patients who took part in the exercise program, had neurotic complaints in addition to depression. Exercise seemed to have a positive effect on different psychosomatic disorders, such as headache, migraine, muscular tension, lumbar pain, obesity, and cardiac neurosis.

Nine of the patients in this study were exercising while using tricyclic antidepressants. The following section will deal with the interaction observed between exercise and medication for these patients, as well as clinical experience based upon other patients studies in the same hospital over the past eight years.

EXPERIENCES WITH EXERCISE
FOR PSYCHIATRIC PATIENTS RECEIVING
PSYCHOPHARMACOLOGICAL TREATMENT

Modum Bads Nervesanatorium is a psychiatric clinic, and it has a population of 106 patients. Most patients have neurotic or character disorders, and very few are psychotic. In the treatment, individual psychotherapy, family therapy and group therapy are emphasized along with occupational and milieu therapy. Psychotropic drugs are used to a limited extent in the treatment of severe depressions, psychoses and sleep disturbances.

Training of aerobic power has been part of the treatment programs since 1975. During these years, many patients have taken part in regular exercise while receiving psychotropic drugs. There have been no dangerous complications observed, such as cardiac diseases, and there have been no episodes of sudden death during exercise. One case of acute dystonia was observed during exercise in a psychotic man who had started receiving antipsychotic medication the day before. This patient experienced acute dystonia while running in the woods, but one can only speculate as to whether or not his dystonia was partly exercise induced.

In the previously reviewed study, 24 patients took part in the training group, and they trained aerobically three times a week for nine weeks. Nine of these patients were receiving tricyclic antidepressant medication in doses varying from 50 to 150 mg/d. Some of the patients complained of common side effects of the medication, such as orthostatism, tachycardia, dry mouth, drowsiness and vertigo, but these side effects did not force them to reduce the intensity of exercise, or drop out of the exercise program.

The effect of exercise on different mental illnesses is being evaluated in an ongoing study. Among the patients, many suffer from somatoform disorders. Patients are taken into the hospital in groups of 8, and they undergo an 8 week program that consists mainly of aerobic exercise and group psychotherapy. More than 70 patients have passed through this program, and about half of them have received tricyclic antidepressants and/or hypnotics. There have been no serious complications observed with the combination of exercise and psychopharmacological treatment.

Patients involved in the research described here have undergone careful medical screening. Patients with a history of cardiovascular disease, or those suspected of having such disease, do not take part in the exercise programs until they have been cleared by a cardiologist. Special care has been taken in exercising patients with coronary heart disease receiving tricyclic antidepressants, even though the literature does not indicate that this is a doubtful combination. The intensity of the training is low, while the doses of medication are increasing. When one has reached steady state level, and the circulation is reasonably well adapted to the medication, intensive exercise can start.

Exercise is a relatively new way of approaching mental illness. It is important when psychiatrists advise patients to exercise, to be reasonably sure that this is medically safe for the patient, so that unnecessary complications can be avoided. If there are too many complications to a new therapeutic approach, the chances for the method to survive and get accepted will be greatly reduced.

SUMMARY

A critical review of the literature regarding the interaction between exercise and medication, shows that our knowledge in this field is limited. The following seems to be reasonably sure: Megadoses (1–3 g/d) of chlorpromazine tend to reduce cardiac output and attenuate the effect of training programs. Therapeutic doses of neuroleptics and tricyclic antidepressant agents often lead to a decrease in blood pressure. The use of beta blockers impair a person's exercise performance, but there are diverging opinions whether or not training effect may be achieved by using them. Exercise induced muscular fatigue and hypoglycemia are common complaints. Physically healthy people who require psychotropic medication, may safely exercise when exercise and medications are titrated under close medical supervision.

PREVENTION AND TREATMENT

7

TENSION REDUCTION WITH EXERCISE

Herbert A. deVries

INTRODUCTION

It has been proposed that relaxation consists of both somatic and cognitive processes, where the former consists of a generalized reduction in activation levels of multiple physiological systems such as the relaxation response of Beary and Benson (1974); and the latter is a more specific pattern of changes superimposed upon this general reduction. Considerable evidence supports such a conceptual framework (Blumenthal, Schocken, Needels and Hindle, 1982; deVries and Adams, 1972; Eysenck, 1975; Schwartz, Davidson, and Goleman, 1978). Indeed, Eysenck (1975) suggests three quite distinct and measurable aspects for the measurement of emotional states: 1) physiological, 2) introspective assessment, and 3) behavioral assessment. While the relationships among the different physiological measurements may be considerable (Gellhorn, 1958; Lader, 1975; Wallace, and Benson, 1972), the relationship between physiological and cognitive measures may be small (Mandler, Mandler, and Uviller, 1958) to nonexistant (deVries and Adams, 1972). In any event, this chapter will focus on the physiological (somatic) effects of aerobic exercise in bringing about a reduction in neuromuscular tension levels.

THEORETICAL BASIS

Physical educators and coaches have long contended that exercise relieves undue resting neuromuscular tension which is one of the better non-invasive measures of the anxiety-tension state (Gellhorn, 1958; Gellhorn and Loofbourrow, 1963; Jacobson, 1938). However, until recently, subjective impression has been the only support for this hypothesis one can, however, justify the testing of this hypothesis on any one or combination of the following physiological bases.

Temperature Effect

Experimental work on cats (Von Euler and Soderberg, 1957) has shown that small temperature rises (such as occur during aerobic exercise) in appropriate structures of the brain stem or the whole body result in decreased muscle spindle activity and synchronized electrical activity in the cortex. Both of these responses are typical of a more relaxed state.

Reduction in Circulating Catecholamines

One of the effects of aerobic conditioning is a significant reduction of circulating catecholamines (Cousineau, Fergusun, DeChamplain, Gauthier, Cote, and Bourassa, 1977; Hartley, Mason, Hogan, Jones, Kotchen, Mougey, Wherry, Pennington, and Ricketts, 1972a; Hartley, Mason, Hogan, Jones, Kotchen, Mougey, Wherry, Pennington, and Ricketts, 1972b).

Inhibition of Nociceptor Afferents by Activation of Mechanoreceptors

There is considerable evidence that in addition to the familiar reflexogenic projections of the muscle spindle afferents (such as the Golgi Tendon Organ afferents which bring about relaxation), such afferents also give off in the spinal cord collateral branches that exert inhibitory presynaptic effects on nociceptive afferent transmission (Wyke, 1982).

pH Effect on Resting Muscle Tension

Irritability of muscle tissue has long been known to increase with increasing pH and to decrease with lowering pH as occurs in aerobic exercise.

Vagal Reflexes from the Lung

It has been shown that distension of the lung by several methods brings about an inhibition of motor activity in the cat (Ginzel and Eldred, 1970).

Enhanced Endorphin Production

Studies have shown that circulating endogenous opioids are increased after aerobic exercise of moderate intensity both in males (Farrell, Gates, Maksud, and Morgan, 1982) and females (Carr, Bullen, Skrinar, Arnold, Rosenblatt, Beitins, Martin, and McArthur, 1981). However, no effect upon mood changes has been demonstrated (Farrell, et al., 1982; Markoff, Ryan, and Young, 1982). Pilot studies in our own lab were also unsuccessful in blocking the physiological relaxation effect of exercise by Naloxone, but further investigation is needed to rule out this factor.

LITERATURE REVIEW: PHYSIOLOGICAL EVIDENCE WITH RESPECT TO TENSION REDUCTION BY EXERCISE

Electromyographic Evidence

Jacobson (1938) was the first to apply EMG techniques to objectively measure nervous tension. In 1936, in a retrospective study, he showed that athletes were better able to relax than non-athletes (Jacobson, 1936).

In 1965, using EMG techniques similar to those of Jacobson, I reported on a prospective pilot study in which 8 subjects had reduced levels of neuro-muscular activity after a 30 minute ride on a bicycle ergometer at a light work-load. The changes were small as might have been expected in normal young subjects and the reduction did not achieve significance (deVries, 1965).

To better test this hypothesis while still using normal subjects, 29 physical education students visited our laboratory on two consecutive days (deVries, 1968). On one day they exercised at bench stepping for five minutes, and on the other day they acted as their own controls. The electrical activity in the right elbow flexor group had a mean decrease of 58% on the exercise day compared with 1.5% on the control day, and this difference was statistically significant ($p < .05$).

To evaluate the chronic effects of physical exercise, 18 members of our faculty conditioning group and seven controls, who maintained a constant level of physical activity, were tested and retested during a period when the experimental subjects had 17 workouts of weight training and interval running. During this period the controls increased their tension levels by 24%, and the experimental subjects decreased theirs by 25% ($p < .02$).

These two experiments both provided statistically significant results favoring a tranquilizer effect for exercise. In the experiment that involved measurement of the acute effect, the subjects had an unexpected anticipatory EMG response on the exercise day. The preexercise levels of electrical activity were considerably higher on the exercise day, which might be considered a flaw in the experimental design.

For this and other reasons, another experiment was set up that provided a more powerful test of the hypothesis. Ten elderly subjects were selected from 60 volunteers who considered themselves to have anxiety-tension problems. All ten subjects showed EMG evidence of residual neuromuscular tension. The following treatment effects were tested: 1) exercise (walking type) at a heart rate of 100 beats/min, 2) the same exercise at a heart rate of 120 beats/min, 3) 400 mg of meprobamate, 4) 400 mg of lactose (placebo), and 5) control. Each subject received each treatment on three occasions.

The tranquilizer drug and placebo were administered double-blind and the anticipatory effect was eliminated by deciding on the treatment for any given day by chance and only after the pre-test data had been recorded. The differences among treatments were significant ($p < .001$), and paired analysis showed that exercise at a heart rate of 100 beats/min lowered electrical activity by 20%, 23%, and 20% at 30, 60 and 90-min following the pre-test. These changes were significantly different from controls (p < .01), but neither the meprobamate nor placebo treatments differed significantly from the control. Exercise at 120 beats/min evoked similar effects, but these differences were not statistically significant. We concluded that, at least in single doses, exercise of an appropriate type and intensity had a significantly greater effect on the resting musculature than did meprobamate, which was one of the most frequently prescribed tranquilizer drugs at that time. More recent work by Sime (1977) has demonstrated a significant reduction in muscle action potential after 12 minutes of treadmill exercise at a light workload (HR 100–110).

Negative findings have also been reported (Balog, 1983; Farmer, Olewine, Comer, Edwards, Coleman, Thomas, and Hames, 1978), but in both cases muscle sampling was from the frontalis muscle. Unfortunately, the frontalis muscle apparently is the muscle of choice for mental stress and headache research, but it is a poor choice if generalizations are to be made to the state of the organism as a whole. In factor analytic studies, Balshan (1962) and Nidever (1959), evaluating the generality of resting muscle tension (EMG) in 16 and 23 muscles respectively of the upper body, found a strong generality to exist among all but 3 muscles of which the frontalis was one. This uniqueness of the frontalis may be related to the fact that it apparently is devoid of muscle spindles (Voss, 1971).

In the interest of decreasing the likelihood of Type II errors in future EMG evaluation of resting neuromuscular tension, the Following suggestions for surface EMG are made:

1. Instrumentation must provide (a) a sensitivity of at least 0.3–0.5 uV/cm (deVries, Burke, Hopper, and Sloan, 1976; Jacobson, 1938), (b) a minimum frequency response of 10–200 Hz measured to the 3dB point (Davis, 1959; Hayes, 1960; Lindstrom and Broman, 1974; Zipp, 1978.
2. A Faraday cage is essential to meet the sensitivity requirement.
3. The muscle of choice for sampling, for purposes discussed here, is the elbow flexor group (Balshan, 1962; deVries, et al., 1976; Jacobson, 1938; Nidever, 1959.
4. Since the tension level of a well relaxed subject (electronically silent) cannot be reduced, it is imperative that tense subjects be employed, or responses to stressful situations be studied.

Hoffman Reflexes

Electrical stimulation of a mixed nerve under appropriate conditions results in two easily measured muscle action potentials. The first to appear (M wave) is the response to the stimulus, which is transmitted directly to the limb muscles via the efferent nerve fibers. The second response (H wave) appears about 20 msec later and is the expression of a monosynaptic reflex, which runs in afferents from the muscle and back again through efferents of the same muscle. Because no internuncial neurons are involved, the size of the second action potential provides a measure of motoneuron excitability under a variety of experimental and pathological conditions (Angel and Hofmann, 1963). After plotting the stimulus-response curves, the amplitude of the largest obtainable H wave is divided by that of the M wave at supramaximal stimulus strength to obtain the H/M ratio (Angel and Hofmann, 1963).

In one experiment (deVries, Wiswell, Bulbulian, and Moritani, 1981), ten subjects were tested three times before and after exercise, and three times before and after a control period of quiet sitting. Exercise consisted of 20 minutes work on a cycle ergometer with the load adjusted to elicit a heart rate 40% between resting and maximal values. Testing consisted of electrical stimulation of the tibial nerve in the popliteal fossa to elicit Hoffmann's reflexes (H waves) and directly transmitted waves (M waves). The H/M ratio was calculated by the Angel and Hofmann method (Angel and Hofmann, 1963). We tested the reliability of this method in our laboratory by ten test-retests on one subject in one day. The coefficient of variation for these data was 9.3%. Biological variability was evaluated post hoc with correlations between 21 paired sets of repeated data showing $0.83 < r < .97$.

We compared the mean of the change in H/M ratio for the three exercise days with the mean change for the three control days. all ten of the subjects showed a fall in the H/M ratio after exercise with an average decrease of 18.2%. On the control days, six of ten subjects showed a small rise, and four showed a small drop, which in no case approached the decrease on the exercise day ($\overline{X} = +1.2\%$). The difference in these responses was statistically significant ($t = 5.64$; $p < .001$).

Achilles Tendon Reflexes

The strength and briskness of tendon jerk reflexes have been routinely used for more than a century to assess the excitability of the central nervous system. However, this approach has only been evaluated recently as a quantitative test through plotting stimulus-response curves in which the stimulus is measured by use of an accelerometer, and the response is the amplitude of the muscle action potential elicited.

In another experiment (deVries, Simard, Wiswell, Heckathorne, and Carabetta, 1982), we examined the effect of exercise on the response to mechanically induced monosynaptic spinal reflex responses by measured tendon taps to the achilles tendon. Six young, healthy, asymptomatic subjects were tested on two days before and after exercise and on two other occasions before and after an equivalent control period of rest to measure the change in their reflex responses to mechanical stimulation. The mean depression of response after exercise was 15.3% ($p < .05$). Changes on the control day were consistently higher.

Catecholamine Effects

The findings of reduced plasma catecholamine after training in three different investigations by two laboratories has been pointed out in the previous section (Cousineau, et al., 1977; Hartley, et al., 1972a; Hartley, et al., 1972b).

Heart Rate

In an experiment comparing the effects of treadmill exercise, meditation and a placebo, Sime found that exercise produced a significantly greater decrease in resting HR than either of the other treatments (Sime, 1977).

Electrodermal Response

In the same investigation referred to under "Heart Rate", Sime also found the exercise effect on the electrodermal response to stress significantly greater than that for meditation or placebo (Sime, 1977).

Relationship of Emotional Stability to Physical Fitness

Two investigations, one retrospective (Cattell, 1960) and one prospective (Young and Ismael, 1976), have shown a positive association between various measures of physical fitness and emotional stability.

SUMMARY

A close examination of the available data suggests substantial agreement among investigators that exercise provides a "tranquilizer" effect. The evidence comes from several different methodological approaches: electromyography, Hoffman Reflex studies, achilles tendon dose-response curves, plasma catecholamine changes, autonomic system changes in heart rate and electrodermal responses to stress, and both retrospective and prospective investigations relating emotional stability to physical fitness. Evidence has also been provided which suggests that appropriate types, intensities, and durations of exercise may be at least equal to and possibly more effective than other modalities such as meditation and pharmacological interventions. The evidence suggests a chronic as well as an immediate effect, and this effect has been found in young, middle aged, and elderly subjects.

Further investigation is needed to elucidate: 1) the physiological mechanisms and site of actions, 2) dose-response relationships, 3) time course of the response, 4) relation of cognitive to somatic parameters of measurement, and 5) relation of measurements under resting conditions to those under stress.

8

REDUCTION OF STATE ANXIETY FOLLOWING ACUTE PHYSICAL ACTIVITY

William P. Morgan

OVERVIEW

Most of the research dealing with the affective beneficience of vigorous physical activity has relied upon chronic interventions. The length of these training programs has typically ranged from six to eight weeks on up to twenty months. Alterations in depression, trait anxiety, and self-esteem have often been reported in these investigations, but in some instances there has not been improvement noted (Morgan, 1984, 1985). The most likely explanation for this inconsistency in the chronic literature stems from the observation that test subjects in the aforementioned studies have often scored within the normal limits to begin with. Hence, one would not expect to observe changes in depression or anxiety if the participants were normal initially. As a matter of fact, it appears that consistent changes have only been observed where individuals have been characterized by moderate affective disturbances from the outset (Morgan, 1984, 1985). There has been far less attention paid to the consequences of acute physical activity. This is important since it is possible that acute changes may occur in the absence of chronic changes, and the present chapter is restricted to an evaluation of acute changes in state anxiety following physical activity, non-cultic meditation, and "time-out" or distraction therapy.

It has been reported by Pitts (1971) that 10 million Americans suffer from anxiety neurosis, and 10–30% of all patients treated by general practitioners are anxiety neurotics. It has also been reported by Pitts that 30–70% of all patients treated by general practitioners and internists have medical conditions based on unrelieved stress. Furthermore, in a recent study of 1,750 primary care physicians it was reported that 85% of the physicians surveyed prescribed exercise for the treatment of depression, and 60% prescribed exercise for the management of anxiety (Ryan, 1983). The exercise mode employed by these respondents consisted of walking, swimming, cycling, strength training, and running.

Walking was the most frequently prescribed form of exercise (i.e., 97%), and running was prescribed the least (i.e., 46%). The extent to which acute physical activity is associated with reduction in state anxiety will be examined next.

EXPERIMENT 1

In view of the fact that walking is the most frequent form of exercise prescription (Byrd, 1963; Ryan, 1983), we evaluated state anxiety in healthy, young, adult males and females following a 17 minute walk (i.e., 1 mile) at grades of zero and five percent. Results were compared with those of control subjects who rested in the supine position for the same length of time. The heart rate responses to the control, 0% grade, and 5% grade walks were 73, 126, and 144 bpm for the women, and 69, 111, and 125 bpm for the men. State anxiety was found to be similar following the three treatments for men and women alike, and it is possible that exercise intensities in the light to moderate range do not reduce state anxiety. Another possibility is that individuals scoring within the normal range on state anxiety do not experience reductions in state anxiety following acute physical activity. Indirect support for this view is provided by Sime (1977) who also noted that state anxiety is not influenced by light exercise.

EXPERIMENT 2

In the next experiment, 40 adult males completed the state form of Spielberger's State-Trait Anxiety Inventory (Spielberger, Gorsuch, & Lushene, 1970) before, immediately following, and 20–30 minutes following 45 minutes of aerobic exercise at approximately 70% of $\dot{V}O_2$ max. A significant reduction (P < .001) in state anxiety was observed at 20–30 minutes following exercise in this group of middle-aged males (Morgan, 1973).

EXPERIMENT 3

The findings observed in the previous experiment were replicated with another group of 15 adult males who completed the state form of the STAI before, 5 minutes following, and again 20–30 minutes following a vigorous 15-minute run. Significant reductions in state anxiety were observed in both post-exercise settings (Morgan, 1973).

EXPERIMENT 4

In the next experiment 28 adult males exercised to complete exhaustion at 80% of their $\dot{V}O_2$ max in the walking and running modes on two separate days. The duration of the exercise bouts averaged 23 and 24 minutes respectively for the running and walking trials. Blood lactate and catecholamine levels were evaluated before and following exercise in this experiment. Blood lactate increased from a mean value of 10 mg% at rest to 90 mg% following both trials. Plasma epinephrine increased fourfold, and plasma norepinephrine increased sevenfold in these experiments. The four-item state anxiety scale was administered before, during, and following these exercise trials on the treadmill. State anxiety increased in linear fashion during the first half of both trials, became asymptotic during the second half of the bout, and decreased significantly immediately following exercise (Morgan, Horstman, Cymerman, and Stokes, 1980).

EXPERIMENT 5

This experiment involved an additional sample of 28 adult males, and the same protocol described in Experiment 4 was utilized. The biochemical and state anxiety findings of the previous experiment were replicated, with the results being nearly identical (Morgan et al., 1980).

EXPERIMENT 6

In the next experiment, Bahrke and Morgan (1978) evaluated the state anxiety of 75 adult males who were randomly assigned to one of three treatments. The treatments consisted of walking on a treadmill at 70 percent of $\dot{V}O_2$ max for 20 min, 20-minutes of non-cultic meditation (Benson's relaxation response), or quiet rest in a sound-filtered room for 20 minutes. The exercise and meditation groups both experienced significant decreases in state anxiety as expected, and the results are summarized in Figure 1. It will be noted, however, that the control group (i.e., placebo) also experienced a reduction in anxiety, and this unexpected change did not differ from results observed for the treatment groups. This finding has led us to propose that "time-out" or "distrac-

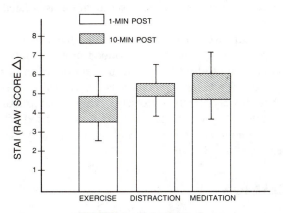

FIGURE 1   State anxiety decrease

tion" from the cares and worries of the day may represent the crucial factor in tension reduction following such diverse treatments as exercise, meditation, and biofeedback.

EXPERIMENT 7

The next experiment was designed in an effort to quantify the extent to which reductions in anxiety remain suppressed following acute physical activity. In this investigation, Seemann (1978) evaluated adult males and females on state anxiety before, immediately following, and again at selected intervals across 24-hours. This research corroborated the previous observation of decreased anxiety following exercise for both men and women. Both groups, however, experienced an increase in state anxiety to the pre-exercise level within 2–4 hours following exercise, and the state anxiety remained stable across the ensuing 20 hours. In other words, the anxiety reduction was transitory, and the tension reduction lasted for approximately 2–4 hours.

WORK IN PROGRESS

We have recently completed a series of experiments dealing with the reduction of state anxiety and blood pressure following (1) exercise, (2) time-out therapy, and (3) warm showers (Raglin & Morgan, in review). This research has served to replicate and extend our earlier experimentation in that state anxiety has been consistently observed to decrease following both acute physical activity and "time-out" therapy, and the effects have been noted to be equivalent for the two treatments. These observed decrements in state anxiety, however, do not exceed those notes for subjects following warm showers lasting 5 minutes. This more recent work supports the view that distraction or "time-out" may be the crucial ingredient in these diverse treatments. In this context, a related report by Wilson, Berger, and Bird (1981) suggests that the anti-anxiety effects of exercise do not exceed those associated with eating a meal!

Our more recent work has extended the earlier experimentation in two ways. First, psychic (STAI) and somatic (blood pressure) dimensions of state anxiety have been examined, and second, the persistence of observed changes has been quantified. While these results must be viewed as preliminary, it appears that the anti-anxiety effects of exercise, while equal to those observed for "time-out" treatments, appear to persist for a longer period of time. This tendency applies to both blood pressure, as well as state anxiety measured with the STAI (Spielberger, et al., 1970).

CONCLUSION

On the basis of the experiments reviewed in this paper it is concluded that acute physical activity of a vigorous nature is *associated* with a decrement in state anxiety, and this tension reduction persists for approximately 2–4 hours. It is unclear at this point as to *why* the tension reduction occurs following exercise, and one hypothesis is that *distraction* from stress-provoking factors plays an important role in this process. There are, of course, viable physiological explanations for the affective beneficience associated with acute physical activity, and these views are addressed elsewhere in the present volume.

9

PSYCHOLOGICAL EFFECTS OF EXERCISE IN THE MIDDLE YEARS

A. H. Ismail

INTRODUCTION

There is a large amount of literature dealing with the psychological effect of exercise. By and large, contradictory results have been reported which are often difficult to interpret because of the complex nature of the phenomenon under consideration. This complexity has resulted in considerable inconsistencies among studies with regard to both internal and external validity. The methodological difficulties associated with studies which deal with the relationship between exercise and personality have been clarified by Morgan (1979) and Eysenck et al. (1982).

Recently emphasis has been devoted to the utilization of multivariate statistical approaches rather than the traditional univariate procedures which assume independence between variables of interest. The use of multivariate procedures enables the researcher to acknowledge the multidimensional nature of exercise as a "natural medicine" not only for physiological benefits but also for psychological health. In order to adequately appreciate the significance of these methodological changes, it is valuable to reflect on how the study of personality and exercise has changed over the years, and how this change has led towards a gradual recognition of the multivariate complexity of personality.

PERSONALITY

Psychometric Approaches

Since ancient times, the study of personality has flourished, guided largely by the intuitive and subjective assessments of philosophers, laymen and researchers. The lack of a precise instrument for the assessment of personality

Appreciation is expressed to Wojtek Chodzko-Zajko and Patrick O'Connor for their help in the preparation of this chapter.

has, and to a large extent still does, hinder the progress of research in this area. The wide variety of personality measures and their often subjective test construction has imposed severe limitations on subsequent research utilizing such instruments.

Initially, exercise scientists tended to restrict their research to studies relating personality to various sports activities (Berger and Littlefield, 1969; Kroll and Carlson, 1967; Whiting and Stembridge, 1965), motor achievement (Schendel, 1965), and physical fitness (Jetté, 1971; Tillman, 1965). By and large, these studies have been limited to adolescents or sportsmen at or near the peak of their careers (Morgan, 1970; Morgan and Hammer, 1974; Morgan and Pollock, 1977). Relatively, few studies have concentrated on middle-aged populations. At Purdue University, emphasis have been devoted to studying the relationships between exercise and personality characteristics of non-athletic adult populations.

Cattell (1970) has provided strong scientific support for the adoption of multivariate factor analytic techniques in the study of personality. Despite this sound theoretical base, most research in the area of personality and exercise has persisted in utilizing statistical techniques which are univariate in nature. Univariate procedures assume independence among variables and thus are limited with regard to their utility when studying complex phenomena such as personality. Consequently our research has emphasized the multivariate approach when studying the relationship between exercise and personality characteristics.

Ismail and Young (1973) compared the relationships between physical fitness and personality characteristics (16PF) in high and low fit subjects before and after a four month physical fitness program. While univariate approaches were successful in differentiating between the high and low fitness groups, these approaches assume independence among the 16 factors and such assumptions are not met as evidenced by the work of several researchers in this area (Kroll and Carlson, 1967, Cattell et al., 1970). Consequently, our data were also analyzed by multivariate approaches which were not only capable of discriminating between the two fitness groups but also provided discriminant function coefficients which reflected the relative importance of each factor involved. Most importantly, the multivariate procedures acknowledged the existence of complex interrelationships among the 16 factors.

In addition to the univariate versus multivariate debate, a good deal of controversy has been generated by the question of "state" versus "trait" approaches to personality measurement. In an important paper, Morgan (1980) advocated the discontinuation of the argument about the value of trait versus state theories. We have systematically investigated relationships between state and trait dimensions of personality at different hierarchical levels (Ismail and Young, 1976).

Our study investigated the relationship between physical fitness and trait personality (16PF) variables at second and third order factor analytic solutions. Factor scores were computed for each subject on each of five second order factors and these data were factor analyzed to extract the third order solutions. The second order factors closely resembled Cattell's factors (Gorsuch and Cattell, 1967). However, subtle differences were observed between initial and final factor structures which may have been due to the influence of the fitness program. The hierarchical third order factor structures appeared to be comparable to the scales of Eysenck. Thus, the 16PF and EPI should not be regarded as contrasting approaches to the measurement of personality but rather the scales are similar but representing different hierarchical levels. In a subsequent study, we combined an established measure of 'state' personality (MAACL, Zuckermann) with more traditional 'trait' measures (16PF, EPI). At the hierarchical level of analysis it was found that state and trait variables do not in fact measure independent aspects of behavior but rather are highly related, (Young and Ismail, 1977). Thus the results of both of these studies are in complete agreement with Morgan's conclusion concerning the trait versus state debate (1980).

Biochemical Correlates of Psychometric Measures

It is not feasible to review even the studies we have carried out at Purdue, let alone make an attempt to comprehensively review the literature from other sources. It is possible however to note several general themes that link the majority of studies in the area of exercise and personality. Repeatedly, studies have shown regular exercise to be associated with favorable changes in emotional health (Ismail and Young, 1973, 1976, 1977, Young and Ismail, 1976). These findings are broadly consistent with those of other researchers (Folkins et al., 1972, Kavanagh et al., 1975, Morgan et al., 1971, Brown et al., 1978 and Greist et al., 1978). deVries and Adams (1972), for instance, compared a bout of moderate exercises with pharmacologic treatment for anxiety-tension states in middle-aged and older subjects and found that exercise had a significantly greater effect upon the resting musculature than meprobamate. Johnson and Spielberger (1968) found that relaxation training significantly reduced anxiety state; similarly, Jetté (1971) found that habitual exercisers were less anxious than non-exercisers.

Not all researchers report antidepressant or anxiolytic effects of exercise, (Morgan, 1979). However, even in these studies the majority of subjects subjectively reported a sense of "exhilaration" and "feeling better" following physical activity. The authors speculate that insignificant results in the study of exercise related changes in personality may often be a function of the insensitivity of many psychometric instruments to the subtle changes which can be expected in psychologically normal subjects.

Whereas psychometric data alone may not be sufficiently sensitive to pick up exercise mediated changes in personality (Koleta, 1979, Koleta et al., 1979), our research has consistently shown that psychometric data can be combined with physiological and biochemical variables to provide a multidimensional interpretation of exercise induced changes in personality. Such approaches not only augment the power of psychometric variables but also represent a biological validation of psychometric instruments while remaining faithful to the natural complexity of personality (Young and Ismail, 1976, Ismail and Young, 1977, 1979).

As yet, our understanding of the biochemical correlates of personality is still extremely limited. The majority of studies have restricted themselves to demonstrating the existence of associations between behavior and measured fluctuations in hormones, neurotransmitters and other psychoactive substances (Mason et al., 1968, 1968, Mason et al., 1968, Heaman et al., 1970, Koch et al., 1974, Jenkins et al., 1969, Rahe et al., 1971, Sloan et al., 1961, Rose et al., 1972, Lobstein et al., 1983). Given our current level of sophistication, it will be a considerable time before we are able to address the issue of what mechanisms underlie these observed associations. Nonetheless, I have no doubt that the study of biochemical correlates is central to the understanding of behavior and accordingly any future investigations in the area of personality and exercise must take these variables into consideration.

Trends in Future Research

With regard to the exercise paradigm, almost no emphasis has been placed on the evaluation of the biochemical correlates of personality. An example of the rare studies conducted along this line is the one completed by Lobstein (1983) who investigated the influence of exercise training on changes in circulating levels of beta endorphin and personality characteristics of middle-aged men. He concluded that there is a "psychobiological" interaction involving physical fitness condition, beta-endorphin levels and emotional stability. At Purdue University, our research has concentrated on the biochemical correlates of depression in normal individuals, and more recently, clinical subjects have been studied as well. In a recent study (Ismail and Sothmann, 1983), we investigated the effects of regular exercise on catecholamine secretion in normal middle aged adults. Catecholamines have received much attention in recent years as psychoactive variables implicated in the regulation of affective disorders (Schildkraut, 1965, Frankenhaeuser, 1970). In our study we investigated epinephrine (E), norepinephrine (NE), metenephrine (MET) and 3methoxy-4hydroxyphenlglycol (MHPG) secretion both at rest and during a normal working day before and after a period of physical training. Our findings reveal that high fit individuals can be differentiated from low fit individuals on the basis of a combination of biochemical (MHPG) and psychometric (MMPI- scale) variables.

These data are encouraging because they suggest that biochemical variables implicated in psychiatric depression may be sensitive to modification by exercise training. In order to adequately test this hypothesis it is necessary to extend our research to clinical patients. We are currently engaged in a preliminary investigation studying the effect of exercise on the personalities of normal and clinically depressed individuals using psychometric variables supplemented by the Dexamethasone Suppression Test (DST) and catecholamine data. Carroll

(1982) has shown cortisol hypersecretion following dexamethasone inhibition to be significantly related to certain subtypes of depressive disorder. In a previous study (White, Ismail and Bottoms, 1975), we have shown cortisol secretion to be sensitive to modification by physical training. Accordingly, it is of particular interest to investigate whether exercise effects on cortisol levels can have any effect on the dexamethasone suppression test in either normal or clinical subjects.

In this paper I have deliberately refrained from concentrating on the results of specific studies. Rather, I have attempted to focus on changing trends in the study of personality. I am convinced that the multidisciplinary study of the biochemical correlates of personality offers much potential for expansion. There is every reason to believe that studying the interactions between exercise and personality will contribute greatly not only to our understanding of the multivariate nature of personality, but also to exercise as preventive medicine.

10

EXERCISE INTERVENTION WITH DEPRESSED OUTPATIENTS

John H. Greist

INTRODUCTION

Depression is the most common mental disorder. Several careful studies done in different American communities have found that 5 percent of the population can be diagnosed as having major depression at any one point in time. At least 10 percent of the population will experience a major depression during their lifetime (some researchers find rates up to 25 percent). Studies in many countries and cultures and across all social classes show a similar frequency of depression. People with a history of serious depression have on the average about five episodes during their lifetime although the number of episodes varies greatly and some people will have only a single episode while others may have many more. At most, half of the people with depression presently receive treatment and some 15 percent of people with major depression will end their lives by suicide. Availability and use of effective antidepressant treatments should lower both morbidity and mortality associated with depression.

Some depressions pass rather quickly without treatment. For mild depression where other aspects of the individual's life are in good order (relationships, job, health, etc.), two kinds of regular psychotherapy are likely to be of benefit (Beck, Rush, Shaw, and Emergy, 1979; Klerman, Rounsaville, Chevron, Neu, and Weissman, 1979). But sometimes even with mild depression, commonly with moderate depression and almost always when depression is severe, antidepressant medication is needed to initiate and maintain a remission. A combination of psychotherapy and antidepressant medication may be the most effective treatment available for nonpsychotic depressions. With psychotic depression, electroconvulsive therapy (ECT) remains the treatment of choice and if antide-

This work was done in collaboration with Marjorie H. Klein, Ph.D., Alan Gurman, Ph.D., Roger R. Eischens, M.S., and Dean Lessor, M.S. and was supported, in part, by grants from the University of Wisconsin Medical School Research Fund, The Wisconsin Alumni Research Foundation, Roche Pharmaceuticals and The National Institutes of Mental Health (MH25546).

pressant medications are to be tried, they must be combined with antipsychotic medications. Psychotherapies are ineffective for psychotic depression.

Many individuals are fearful about taking psychotropic medications and others are unwilling to participate in psychotherapy. Medications also have annoying side effects, psychotherapies are costly and ECT usually requires hospitalization.

PERSONAL EXPERIENCE

As a student athlete, I was dimly aware of the mood elevating effects of many training sessions. When called among the tasks of real life I grew to appreciate the way exercise lysed anxiety and anger as well as lifting mood. Other adult athletes reported similar reactions to exercise and, as the care of depressed patients became my responsibility, I noted that many of them were physically unfit. I also learned that some people became severely depressed even while exercising.

A review of the literature available in 1975 uncovered a few studies suggesting that exercise had mood-elevating properties in clinically well individuals who nevertheless scored in the depressed range on self-report depression questionnaires (McPherson, Paivio, Yuhasz, Rechnitzer, Pickard, and Lefcoe ,1967; Morgan, Roberts, Brand, and Feinerman, 1970; Folkins, Lynch, and Gardner, 1972). Several of my depressed patients who began regular exercise responded with prompt and clear remissions. Other patients, often those most severely ill, failed to improve and many patients were unable to adhere to a regular exercise program.

FIRST WISCONSIN STUDY

Intrigued with these clinical observations and aware of the variable results and high costs of psychotherapies and the annoying side effects of antidepressant medications, I wanted to study the possible antidepressant effects of exercise in a clinically depressed population. Marjorie Klein, Alan Gurman and I were conducting a controlled trial of two kinds of psychotherapy for patients with moderate depression and it became possible to add exercise as another treatment condition. Despite reluctance of some colleagues to place patients at a risk of such heretical treatment, we were able to conduct a random assignment study of patients whose chief complaint was depression, who scored at or above the 65th percentile on the depression cluster of the Symptom Checklist 90 (SCL-90) (Derogatis, Lipman, and Covi, 1973) and whose depression caused substantial interference with performance of their major life role. Exercise, in the form of walking and jogging, proved to be at least as effective as both kinds of psychotherapy at the completion of treatment and at follow-up (see Figure 1) (Greist, Klein, Eischens, Faris, Gurman, and Morgan, 1979).

Many questions remained unanswered: Could the antidepressant effect of exercise be replicated? What kinds of depression are responsive to exercise?

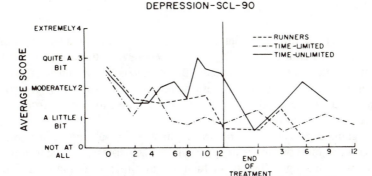

FIGURE 1 Depression scores of patients treated with running only, and with two kinds of psychotherapy. Time-limited psychotherapy consisted of ten behaviorally focused sessions. Time-unlimited psychotherapy was dynamic, insight-oriented psychotherapy.

Would combinations of exercise and psychotherapy or medications or all three be better than exercise alone? What dose of exercise is required for an antidepressant effect? What mechanisms underlie any antidepressant effect of exercise? Why do some depressed individuals fail to respond to exercise? In our view, exercise treatment remained experimental and we felt it important to learn what we could from the experience of other researchers and to continue our research on the effectiveness of exercise in the treatment of clinical depression.

Since anxiety and depression covary so strongly, and the clinical differentiation of anxiety and depressive disorder is sometimes difficult (Lipman, 1982; Mountjoy and Roth, 1982), studies showing reduction in anxiety with exercise (Karbe, 1966; deVries, 1968; Popejoy, 1968; Hanson, 1971; Morgan, 1979; Young, 1979) may also be relevant to the possible antidepressant effects of exercise. One case study (Blue, 1979) and one group study (Kavanagh, Shepard, Tuck and Quereshi, 1977), although somewhat lacking in control procedures, found positive outcomes for jogging programs with clinically depressed populations. Two doctoral dissertations were also of interest. A study of 17 depressed outpatients who were randomly assigned to treatment with cognitive behavior therapy (n = 6), jogging (n = 5) and a waiting list control group (n = 6) found that both cognitive behavior therapy and jogging treatment were significantly more effective than the control procedure in reducing Beck Depression Inventory scores (Hess-Homeier, 1981). The other study involved 7 clinically depressed male and female outpatients assessed with the Depression Adjective Checklist (DACL) studied in an A.B.A.B. single-subject design for a six-week period. While the entire group failed to achieve statistically significant differences (p < .08), 3 subjects showed significant differences while 4 did not (Hartz, 1982).

SECOND WISCONSIN STUDY

Because of difficulty obtaining referral of clinical subjects from colleagues convinced of the primacy of psychotherapy in the treatment of depression, we elected to recruit volunteers from the community through newspaper advertisements. These subjects were generally well matched with new clinic patients with one exception: They had often failed to benefit from previous treatment, sometimes in our clinic.

Again, depression or some synonym was the subject's chief complaint, they scored at or above the 65th percentile on the depression cluster of the SCL-90 and were having difficulty in their major life role because of depressed mood. Subjects all met Research Diagnostic Criteria for major or minor depression, were not thought to be acutely suicidal or to require immediate treatment with antidepressant medications or electroconvulsive therapy.

Sixty subjects were randomly assigned to exercise (walking and jogging for a total of 12 sessions with "running therapists" and at least 3 sessions weekly alone or with their therapist for 12 weeks), Benson's noncultic relaxation response meditation (12 sessions with therapists and instruction to participate in at least 3 sessions weekly with or without the therapist) and 12 sessions of group psychotherapy provided by two experienced therapists. All therapists provided all treatments (except that two therapists did all the group therapy) to control for possible therapist effect. Symptom change for depression was assessed using the SCL-90 pre, post and at one-, three- and nine-month follow-up (see Figure 2).

This study again found exercise to be significantly effective, both statistically and clinically, for moderate depression. Comparison with a traditional treatment (group psychotherapy) and another cult activity (meditation) showed no significant advantage for any treatment. During follow-up, subjects who had exercised or meditated maintained their improvements while those who had group therapy lost some of their gains.

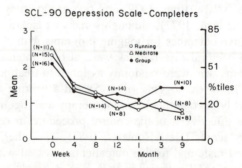

FIGURE 2 Depression scores of volunteer subjects treated with running, meditation, and group therapy.

EXERCISE TECHNIQUE

We chose walking-jogging as our form of exercise because for most people it is convenient and economical. We quickly realized that most exercisers, even when not depressed, fail to comply with an exercise regimen for more than a few weeks. Techniques to increase adherence were carefully though through and described (Eischens, Kane, Wilcox, and Greist, 1979; Eischens and Greist, 1984). Most people starting to run have in their mind's eye an image of Joan Benoit, Gretta Waitz, Allison Roe, Frank Shorter, Bill Rodgers or Alberto Salazar. They push too hard, become fatigued and sore and quickly drop out. The running therapist modeled a more gentle, graduated approach to exercise that was intended to leave subjects looking forward to the next run rather than dreading it.

COMMENT

It now seems likely that exercise has mood-elevating properties for many individuals with clinical depression. Antidepressant exercise needs to be done regularly and for most individuals, three sessions per week is a minimum and more sessions appear advantageous. Exercise has a mood state-elevating effect and also appears to have a mood trait-elevating effect which is more difficult to define because of the self-limiting nature of most depressions.

Adherence to a prescription of exercise remains a limitation of this treatment approach although dropouts are probably no more frequent than for drug or psychotherapies. Providing non-competitive exercise therapists who model comfortable exercise and matching choice of exercise with individual preference seem important elements in enhancing adherence.

Theoreticians often overemphasize one perspective to make a point. Depression has been seen as "endogenous" or arising from a deranged biochemistry and as "reactive" to experiences in the individual's life. Nature being complex, it seems likely that depression is the symptomatic manifestation of multiple etiologic factors expressed through the final common pathway we label depression (Akiskal and McKinney, 1975). Inheritance or genetic predisposition, developmental factors such as early loss of a parent, stress from problems in relationships, physical illness of intense grief all combine to produce the disorder of depression. Each individual has a pattern of genetic, developmental, environmental, social, psychological and physiological characteristics that combine to permit or protect against depression at any point in time. How exercise interferes with or contributes to the development of depression remains an intriguing question. While a good start has been made in finding answers to questions about exercise and mental disorders, a great deal of work remains to be cone on indications for exercise treatment, effective elements in exercise therapies, prescription variables (frequency, duration and intensity), combination of exercise with other treatments, techniques to improve adherence and mechanisms underlying effectiveness.

11

COMPARATIVE EFFECTIVENESS OF RUNNING THERAPY AND PSYCHOTHERAPY

Dorothy V. Harris

INTRODUCTION

Ten billion dollars are spent annually on the treatment of depression in the United States (National Institute of Mental Health, 1981). This fact, coupled with the prospect of one in four Americans experiencing a bout with depression serious enough to warrant medical or psychological assistance at some point during their life (American Psychiatric Association, 1980), makes the search for low cost, effective and accessible treatments a priority. With an increasing awareness of holistic wellness and the belief that physical exercise has a soma-topsychic effect (Harris, 1973), a new dimension has been added to treatment possibilities for depression. Some innovative therapists and sport scientists have used aerobic exercise as a treatment, or as an adjunct to treatment, for mild to moderate depression. Some of the research that has been conducted at The Pennsylvania State University will be cited to illustrate the comparative effectiveness of running therapy and psychotherapy.

STUDY 1

Using the work of Greist, Klein, Eischens, and Faris (1978) as a model, Reuter, Mutrie, and Harris (1984) conducted a similar study using a small student population. Eighteen subjects who had sought help for depression at the mental health clinic of a large university were randomly assigned to one of two treatment groups. After the initial intake interview, subjects were assigned to a counseling therapist and scheduled to meet for at least 30 minutes per week. Counseling therapy may have been individual, group or a combination of the two types. The time spent in counseling therapy was individually determined, therefore subjects may have received varying amounts of therapy before they

TABLE 1   Pre- and post-scores on the Beck Depression Inventory (BDI).

Subjects	Totals	Means	SD
Running group ($n = 9$)			
Pre-BDI	207	23.00	7.58
Post-BDI	46	5.10	4.75
Non-running group ($n = 9$)			
Pre-BDI	208	23.10	11.02
Post-BDI	167	18.56	7.70

Note: Adapted from Reuter (1979).

were considered well enough to be discharged. The counseling therapy was under the direction of professional psychiatrists and psychologists.

Those participating in the running therapy ran under supervision for at least 20 minutes three times per week. No criterion levels for distance or speed were set. The intensity and duration of the run were determined by each subject's physical condition. Throughout the running sessions, proper methods of warm-up and non-competitive running were emphasized.

The pre- and post-Beck Depression Inventory (BDI) scores for running and counseling alone did not differ significantly prior to the running intervention. The post-BDI mean for the running counseling (5.1) was well within normal range. The counseling alone mean was 18.56 on the post-BDI, indicating they were still moderately depressed. (See Table 1 and Figure 1 below).

The results of a two-way analysis of variance with repeated measures contrasting the pre- and post-BDI scores of both groups revealed a significant

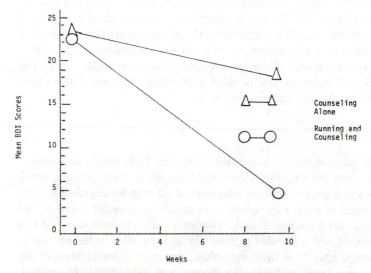

FIGURE 1   Running and counseling therapy versus counseling alone.

interaction effect F (1, 16) = 9.32, p < .01. Post hoc tests of the simple
effects were conducted by the Tukey Wholly Significant Difference method
(WSD), to determine the exact nature of this interaction effect. The between
groups simple effects were not significant at the pre-test, but the difference
between the groups was significant at the post-test. The within group simple
effect was not significant for the counseling alone group, but the differences
between the pre- and post-means for the running and counseling groups were
significant. It would appear from these results that running is an effective adjunct to counseling therapy in the treatment of depression.

STUDY 2

Fremont (1983) expanded on the design used by Reuter et al. (1984). His
study was designed to examine the separate and combined effects of counseling
and aerobic exercise in the treatment of mild and moderate depression. Forty-
nine depressed volunteers (13 males and 36 females) ranging in age from 19–62
were randomly assigned to one of the three treatment conditions. Subjects in the
first condition participated in a supervised, structured running program which
was conducted in small groups and met for 20 minutes three times a week.
Subjects in the second condition met individually with a counselor one hour
each week for cognitively based counseling. Subjects in the third condition
received counseling and also participated in the running program. All treatment
programs were 10 weeks.

All three treatment conditions produced significant but not differential
improvement in self-reports of depression, anxiety and other related mood

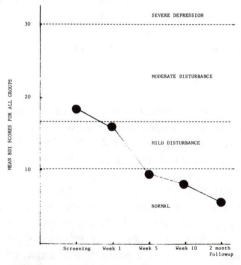

FIGURE 2   Change in depression scores over time.
Fremont (1983).

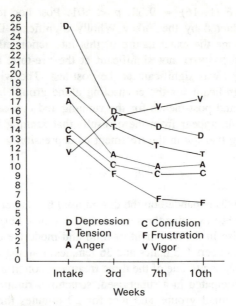

FIGURE 3 Summary of effects. Fremont, 1983.

states. While counseling and running therapies were equally effective, combining both treatments was not more beneficial than either treatment applied separately. It appeared, however, that the initially more anxious, tense and fatigued subjects were more likely to drop out of the running-only condition. Improvement in mood was not related to improvement in physical fitness as measured by the 12-minute walk/run. In fact, it was observed that the most dramatic improvements occurred during the first few weeks of the exercise program (See Figures 2 and 3).

STUDY 3

The effect of regular exercise (10 weeks, 3 times/week) on mood (Profile of Moods Scale, POMS), was compared to members of an English class who served as controls (Mutrie & Harris, 1984). (See Table 2). The experimental group ($n = 14$) was enrolled in a jogging class; the control group ($n = 14$) was not involved in any exercise program. Both groups were tested on the POMS at the beginning, midway through and at the end of the ten weeks.

The MANOVA showed a significant group (jogging, English) X Time (beginning, midway, end) interaction, $F (2, 25) = 4.01$, $p < .03$. There were no other significant MANOVA effects. The subsequent univariate ANOVA's show two of the variables to have significant interaction effects, anger, $F (2, 47) = 3.478$, $p < .04$ and tension, $F (2, 51) = 3.629$, $p < .04$. WSD

TABLE 2 Mean tension and anger scores (POMS).

Mood	Group	Time of term		
		Begin	Midway	End
Anger	Jogging students (n = 14)	9.21	6.57	6.86
	English students (n = 14)	7.36	13.36	8.98
Tension	Jogging students	10.50	7.57	6.79
	English students	12.36	17.00	13.14

Note: Adapted from Mutrie and Harris (1984).

followup tests on the simple effects of the group X time interactions show that the two groups (jogging and English) did not differ significantly at the beginning or end of ten weeks but did differ, $p < .05$, at the midway testing period. The English class also showed a significant increase in anger, $p < .05$, from beginning to the midway point during the ten weeks. The two groups did not differ at the beginning of term on the tension variable, however they did differ ($p < .05$) at both the midpoint and at the end of the ten weeks. The jogging group showed a significant decrease in tension from beginning to end of term ($p < .05$) while the English group showed a significant increase of tension at the midpoint during the ten weeks (See Table 2 and Figure 4). These findings

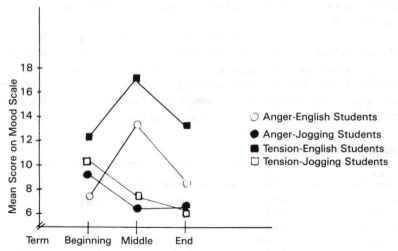

FIGURE 4 Pattern of anger and tension scores (POMS). Mutrie and Harris (1984).

suggest that students who are exercising while they are adjusting to their first term of university study cope more effectively than those who do not have exercise as part of their regular program.

STUDY 4

A study completed by Tooman (1982) is also relevant to the discussion of the influence exercise has on anxiety and moods. The beneficial effects of running were supported indirectly when two groups of runners, competitive ($n = 20$) and recreational ($n = 20$) with similar running histories and capabilities were asked not to run for two days while anxiety and moods were monitored. The testing covered a four day period with the runners reporting for the first session of testing prior to a regular run. Measures on the POMS and the State-Trait Anxiety Inventory (STAI) were taken before and after the run and the subsequent two days without running. These scores are shown on Table 3. On day four the Ss were asked to resume their regular running pattern and report for testing following the run.

The POMS and STAI scores were subjected to a 2 (competitive versus recreational runners) X 5 (testing sessions) analysis of variance with repeated measures. There was a significant main effect for type of runner on state anxiety $F (1, 38) = 6.102, p = < .05$, with the competitive runners being significantly lower. A significant main effect on the anger subscale of the POMS was also observed with the competitive runners being significantly less angry $F (1, 38) = 5.273, p < .05$. The competitive runners had more positive moods on all the subscales of the POMS, however anger was the only significantly different subscale.

The results of this study demonstrate that depriving regular runners of running for only two days increased state anxiety levels, tension and confusion and decreased levels of vigor in both competitive and recreational runners. Further, it was observed that these negative effects of running deprivation disappeared on the resumption of running after a two day lay-off. On day one the measures taken before and after a regular run demonstrated that running led to

TABLE 3 Pre- and post-run mood scores ($n = 40$).

Variable	Scale	Pre-run	Post-run	P
Anger	POMS	4.73	1.95	.01
Confusion	POMS	5.80	4.10	.01
Depression	POMS	6.18	3.70	.01
Fatigue	POMS	6.43	5.33	NS
Tension	POMS	7.45	3.25	.01
Vigor	POMS	17.33	18.48	NS
State anxiety	STAI	34.70	30.52	.01

Note: Adapted from Tooman (1982).

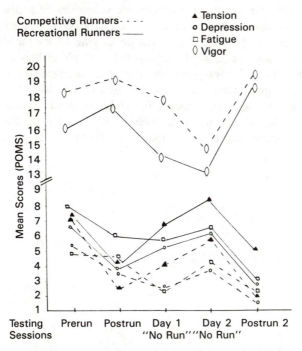

FIGURE 5 Patterns of tension, depression, vigor and fatigue
for competitive and recreational runners. Tooman (1982).

improved mood and reduced anxiety. When comparing the pre-run and post-run
scores, the post-run scores showed significant decreases in tension, depression,
anger, confusion and state anxiety.

COMMENTS

To date several methodological problems exist in the current literature.
Four major design problems limit internal validity:

1. The designs have often lacked no-treatment control conditions which
   would allow the hypothesis of spontaneous remission, without treatment, to be tested.
2. The designs have usually not included testing of the hypothesis that
   running is more than a placebo effect.
3. The effect of exercise has often been confounded with time in contact
   with a professional (a therapist or running leader), with runners often
   receiving more contact time than other groups.
4. The effect of exercise has usually been confounded with the effect of
   contact with a group of runners and running leader.

In addition, the use of subjects who are volunteers or patients in private clinics limits external validity. Furthermore, the process by which exercise may have its effect has not been identified. The underlying theory for using exercise as a treatment in depression would suggest that both physiological and psychological parameters will covary, but much of the completed research has not included physiological parameters. The research to date has, however, generated testable hypotheses. Improvement in aerobic fitness is associated with enhanced mood. The question that remains to be addressed is whether or not this relationship is *causal*, and if so, the mechanism(s) involved.

12

EXERCISE AS AN ADJUNCT TO THE TREATMENT OF MENTAL DISORDERS

Robert S. Brown

INTRODUCTION

The prescription of physical exercise for the treatment of emotional disorders is not a new idea; activity therapy, dance therapy, and recreational therapy have been a part of the inpatient treatment of psychiatric patients for many years. But now its use for outpatients in the office practice of psychiatry is being recommended. The purpose of this chapter is to describe the adjunctive use of exercise therapy in the outpatient care of patients with anxiety and depression, and also to discuss its use in the management of stress associated with such physical disease as renal failure and cancer.

I have prescribed exercise in my practice during the past decade with three different but overlapping groups: 1) college students in a course in mental health; 2) psychiatric patients with a wide range of presenting symptoms; and 3) surgical oncology and renal dialysis-transplantation patients, the latter presenting symptoms of stress that exercise helps relieve. Each group will be discussed both from the perspective of treatment and prevention.

TEACHING MENTAL HEALTH TO COLLEGE STUDENTS WITH THE EXERCISE APPROACH

My method of teaching coping skills to college students was modified to include Lazarus's (1981) elements of coping: 1) information seeking; 2) direct acting, 3) inhibition of action, and 4) intrapsychic processes. I dealt with traditional aspects of stress management in the 16-week semester course I have taught twice a year since 1971 at the University of Virginia. When possible (about a third of the time), I interviewed patients in front of the class with a story-telling format and a question-and-answer period to follow. The objectives of the course were to teach students: 1) selected principles of psychological adjustment to the normal stresses of life; 2) how to develop and maintain a sense of well-being and the ability to tolerate unavoidable discomfort; and 3) how to recognize and deal effectively with depression and anxiety and to consider the possibility that these states might be due to failures in planning, the neglect of commonsense health practices, impaired interpersonal relationships, and/or organ system malfunction. The relevance of this course material to the lives of the students and their families was emphasized. Besides lectures, patient interviews, and guest speakers, movies were provided and small group discussions were led by teaching assistants, and the students were taught ways to improve their own insight and functioning. The basic philosophy of the course rested on the belief that people can learn to face life in courageous and caring ways; that psychological resources can be enriched; that some—perhaps most—stress can be anticipated and prepared for; and that the first step in the process of improving coping strategy is to recognize one's own characteristic way of dealing with stress.*

Self-management techniques taught included both mandatory self-assessment of coping strategies and elective options of exercise, compliance contracts, and exercise partners. About half of the final grade for the course could be earned by self-management options, the most popular of which was the exercise option, which required a minimum of 45 minutes of aerobic exercise at least three days a week for 10 weeks. First- and last-day physical measures taken included resting and post-exercise blood pressure, pulse and respiration rate, height and weight, and the effects of a mile-and-a-half run on an indoor track. Exercise journals that recorded both physical and psychological variables such as mood and significant life events were monitored each week by teaching assistants.

Over the past several years, a data base of approximately 5,000 students in the mental health course was established, confirming my earlier finding (Brown, 1978) that regular exercise is associated with significantly improved general activation and the relief of anxiety and depression. Negative affects such as anger, hostility, fatigue and inertia were significantly decreased, and sleep and dreams improved. Informal follow-up indicates that many students, who had not regularly exercised before, continued to show benefit and improve lifestyles (including exercise) for up to seven years after leaving the mental health course.

In order to encourage students to exercise, I offered: 1) special training sessions on how to exercise, 2) exercise with an assigned student (or patient) once a week for approximately 45 minutes over a period of 10 weeks, 3) a weekly telephone conversation during that time with the assigned exercise partner, and 4) a written critique after each exercise session indicating how the exercise partner had reacted to it. Analysis to date indicates that the exercise

---

*A course syllabus is available on request.

partner elective is an effective method for maintaining an optimal degree of exercise participation.

The compliance elective, the third self-management technique offered, involved a contract signed by both student and instructor, pledging that the student would improve his/her diet, give up tobacco and alcohol, or other specific threats to health. Students were required to keep a pledged journal record of success in complying. Credit was based on an honest, whole-hearted effort to keep the contract, and on maintaining an accurate record of this effort. The compliance journal was combined with a fitness journal, but students could use either or both. Students who recorded compliance fewer than three times a week earned no credit. Many using the compliance program stopped smoking, drank less alcohol, and worked on sensible weight reduction.

EXERCISE AS AN ADJUNCT TO PSYCHIATRIC TREATMENT

The success of the mental health course in helping large numbers of students improve their physical and mental health led to the use of exercise as an adjunct to psychotherapy in my outpatient psychiatric practice. The systematic encouragement of physical exercise among psychiatric patients has not been widely reported, but several reports suggest that it may be efficacious (Brown, 1978; Griest, 1979). Because I continued to modify my method of assessing its benefits, I offer here only a descriptive account of my work, discussing it under three categories: 1) the assessment of psychiatric patients' lifestyles; 2) the prescription of exercise for them; and 3) their acceptance of exercise.

Assessing the Lifestyles of Psychiatric Outpatients

The effects of lifestyle on physical health are thought to be highly significant. "As much as 50% of mortality from the ten leading cause of death in the United States can be traced to lifestyle" (Hamburg, 1982, p. 3). The complex interaction between lifestyle and *mental* health, however, is not yet understood. We do not know what motivates people to adopt and maintain healthy lifestyles. One hypothesis is that psychological problems like frustration, unhappiness, or depression may impair the normal impetus to follow a healthy lifestyle. We have identified few extrinsic factors in low motivation other than poverty and the lack of education or opportunity. In order to understand some of the intrinsic determinants of lifestyle, and to study their interaction with standard measures of psychological functioning, I developed an objective test (Assessment of Operational Mode, Brown, 1983) to give to outpatient psychiatric patients during their initial visit.

It is divided into three sections (Body, Mind, and Spirit), with each section further divided into four parts. The *Body* section measures general fitness, appetite control, tolerance of pain and discomfort, and quality of sleep and rest. The *Mind* section deals with decisions, communication, consideration for others, and regard for truth. The *Spirit* section refers to spiritual concepts and qualities of hope, forbearance, and empathy. The test has been given to college students, funeral directors, and psychiatric outpatients. A total score of more than 12 negative replies identifies people who need counseling for lifestyle change. To date, the test has been readily accepted by people of widely different ages and significantly different socioeconomic levels. Requiring only 36 "yes/ no" statements, it is easily administered and takes little time.

The administration of the lifestyle test was preceded by a study of the self-assessment of college students regarding perception of their physical fitness and physical, emotional, and spiritual health. From the Fall semester of 1980 through the Spring semester of 1983, students were classified according to a five-option descriptive schema (excellent, good, average, fair and poor) to describe their health. The summary of demographic data for the students enrolled in the mental health, course is presented in Table 1. These findings indicated that a lifestyle test would probably be a feasible way to identify specific problems among healthy students, and this observation led to the hypothesis that a lifestyle test for psychiatric outpatients might be expedient and informative.

TABLE 1   Demographic data of students enrolled in mental health

Health status	Fall 1980	Spring 1981	Fall 1981	Spring 1982	Fall 1982	Spring 1983
Physical fitness						
Poor	5	8	2	4	7	13
Fair	17	54	23	44	38	75
Average	73	143	53	126	121	52
Good	122	245	110	179	172	215
Excellent	50	53	45	37	55	40
Physical health						
Poor	1	1	2	1	1	4
Fair	7	24	4	17	13	29
Average	32	79	29	65	68	99
Good	121	264	123	191	204	247
Excellent	95	140	76	120	113	119
Emotional health						
Poor	4	4	3	4	4	7
Fair	16	31	9	21	30	32
Average	64	121	46	88	81	138
Good	122	271	127	205	217	257
Excellent	60	97	49	82	68	60
Spiritual health						
Poor	8	6	1	9	6	10
Fair	17	55	10	27	28	29
Average	72	141	62	101	109	153
Good	114	228	115	192	190	241
Excellent	53	86	37	59	59	55

Note: Number of students reporting status of health.

About a year ago, the lifestyle test was added to a battery of screening tests I give my psychiatric outpatients during their initial visit. The battery includes the following instruments: 1) The Center for the Epidemiological Studies of Depression Test (Weissman, 1980), 2) Spielberger State Anxiety Inventory (Spielberger, 1970), 3) Spielberger Trait Anxiety Inventory, 4) Exercise Inventory (Paffenbarger, 1978), 5) Habits Inventory, and 6) Physical Symptoms Checklist.

As in most psychiatric practices, most patients scored high on anxiety and depression. Few, regardless of their psychiatric diagnosis, took regular exercise or reported being physically fit. Nicotine and ethanol use was common, along with a great variety of physical symptoms. Spiritual factors remain to be analyzed.

The diagnostic interview was conducted after the results of screening psychological tests became available, and followed a story-telling model ("tell me the story of your problem," and "please begin with what you consider to be the beginning of your story"). The patient would be questioned about his/her story, a formal mental status examination was conducted, and diagnosis was made according to DSM-III (Diagnostic and Statistical Manual of the American Psychiatric Association, Third Edition, 1980). When appropriate, a neurological examination and/or diagnostic blood tests were performed. At the conclusion of the diagnostic interview, each patient was given the examiner's diagnostic impression in terms he/she could understand, and, under the circumstances, accept.

Prescribing Exercise for Psychiatric Outpatients

Most patients were eager to learn what they could do to improve their mental health. Some requested medication. Aware of the patient's responses to the screening test, the examiner then reviewed specific steps that might be taken to regain control of his/her life. For most, it was necessary to recommend a hopeful and patient attitude, and to point out that common mental disorders, like depression, are often self-limited and usually abate. The prescription of exercise for mental disorders, like anxiety and depression, fell on deaf ears except when phrased in special terms, incorporated in the treatment plan, and added to traditionally accepted psychiatric treatment. Only in the most severe cases was psychotropic medication prescribed at the outset, then the patient was encouraged to take it along but advised to use it only when necessary. Patients with severe major depressions were usually treated with tricyclic antidepressants, but were also encouraged to exercise.

Acceptance of Exercise among Psychiatric Patients

Although when exercise was made a part of the treatment plan, psychiatric outpatients tended to accept it, their acceptance was influenced by their past experience of exercise, the severity of their illness, their age, and their educational level and socioeconomic status. Young, well-educated adults who previously had positive experience with exercise needed little encouragement to exercise as part of the treatment plan. Among older adults, and those who though of exercise not required by work as frivolous, acceptance was limited. The primary exercise recommended was brisk walking. Anyone who wanted a pocket fitness journal such as we gave mental health students could have one. Patients were encouraged to walk until they could cover a mile in 15 minutes, gradually increasing to three miles a day in 45 minutes. Some patients were given "Walking for Exercise and Pleasure," published by the President's Council on Physical Fitness and Sports. Whenever appropriate, the walking prescription was carried out with the patient during his/her sessions. Exercise partners were assigned to patients who were socially isolated and needed reinforcement. Student volunteers trained and screened for emotional stability formed a cadre of exercise partners.

A few minutes in each treatment session were spent talking over the patient's progress in exercise, reviewing his/her fitness journal, and encouraging compliance. Occasionally, if I forgot to bring up the subject of exercise, patients would be pleased to introduce the topic themselves.

EXERCISE FOR STRESS MANAGEMENT
IN RENAL DIALYSIS AND CANCER

The benefit of exercise in the treatment of coronary artery disease and diabetes mellitus is acknowledged, but its importance as an adjunct to the treatment of other major physical illnesses such as renal failure and cancer has only recently been noted (Goldberg, 1980; Brown, 1984). The hypertension, anemia, and hypertriglyceridemia of renal dialysis patients, who exercise regularly, showed improvement and they obtained psychological benefits like those of exercising healthy subjects. The hazards and risks associated with exercise for dialysis patients are considered less important than the improved mental and physical health exercise promotes. An improved quality of life for selected dialysis patients who exercised has been reported in a limited number of studies (Goldberg, 1980).

Since half the anguish of having cancer arises from the need for emotional and social adjustment to the situation, long-term cancer survivors, and increasingly large population, may be especially susceptible to stress, and will require psychological sensitive physicians and strong social support. Our work at the University of Virginia indicated that they need as much physical activity as can be tolerated (Brown, 1984).

The emotional needs of cancer patients have been studied with the use of battery of screening psychological tests like those used with psychiatric outpatients. Results suggest that as a group, cancer patients are less anxious and depressed than are psychiatric outpatients, but many have a lifestyle that includes little or no regular exercise. When it is prescribed for them, they comply if physically able and if encouraged by their oncologist. The availability of exercise partners promotes compliance. Since maladaptive patterns of behavior, when present in the cancer patient, begin early and tend to persist, it is essential that intervention such as exercise programs be established early in their treatment.

SUMMARY

Exercise may be successfully incorporated into a mental health course to teach coping strategies to college students, and its effects may be long-lasting. Psychiatric outpatients screened with psychological and lifestyle tests will accept exercise when it is part of a legitimate treatment plan. Those who do exercise on a regular basis then show significant improvement in anxiety and depression. Patients on renal dialysis, and those who are long-term survivors of cancer have an improved quality of life when exercise is thoughtfully added to their treatment regimen.

13

STRESS LEVELS IN SWIMMERS

Bonnie G. Berger

INTRODUCTION

It is widely accepted that regular exercise results in a number of physiological benefits. It has been reported by Sharkey (1984), for example, that exercise increases the stroke volume of the heart, reduces blood pressure, and increases high density lipoprotein. Physically active individuals also have greater muscle mass, strength, and muscle tone, along with increases in flexibility and balance as well as a reduced likelihood of osteoporosis (Smith & Serfass, 1981).

Compared to the tangible physiological benefits, the psychological rewards of exercise are more elusive. Regular exercisers "know" that they reap a multitude of psychological benefits (Berger, 1979b). Their testimonies of the values and joys of exercise fill the pages of running magazines. Yet despite these insightful articles, techniques designed to maximize the psychological effects of exertion are still in their infancy (Berger, 1982). For some tentative exercise guidelines designed to enhance psychological well-being, see Berger (1983/1984, 1984b).

Investigating the psychological effects of exercise is beset with problems. The mood changes associated with exercise probably do not remain stable over time (Berger, 1984a; Morgan, 1973), and mood alteration seems to be affected by the exercise conditions (Berger & Owen, 1986). Results of exercising in a laboratory setting may be very different from those occurring in the real world of open fields, crowded streets, or health clubs. Field experiments, although highly desirable, pose a host of practical problems that are nearly impossible to eliminate. Some of the more apparent problems relate to self-selection of subjects, placebo effects, and the availability of subjects for repeated testing.

Despite such problems, the results of several highly disparate studies have led to similar findings. Exercise, or at least running, helps the participant reduce many indices of psychological stress (Berger, 1983/1984, 1986; Berger, Freidmann, & Eaton, in review; Sachs & Buffone, 1984; Sacks & Sachs,

1981). Runners tend to report less anxiety, depression, anger, and confusion, and more vigor (Berger, 1984a; 1984c; Morgan, 1980; Morgan & Pollock, 1977; Wilson, Berger & Bird,1981). Some of the unresolved issues which my colleagues and I have begun to investigate are:

1. Which types of exercise are most conducive to mood elevation?
2. How long should an exercise session continue in order to facilitate psychological benefits?
3. Do exercise participants need to establish a minimal fitness level before psychological benefits can occur?
4. How do the psychological benefits of exercise for women and men in the "normal" population compare with those of individuals exhibiting psychopathology?
5. How effective are the stress reduction benefits of exercise when compared with other treatments such as meditation, psychotherapy, and medication?
6. Does the exercise itself provide the psychological benefits, or are other factors associated with the exercise involved?

Many of these questions are interrelated and difficult to answer unless multivariate paradigms are employed. For example, the answer to the last question may vary as a function of exercise mode (e.g., question 1 above).

EXERCISE MODE: SIMILARITIES OF SWIMMING AND RUNNING

A primary interest of our group has involved the question of whether or not swimming produces psychological benefits similar to those observed for running. Contrary to the belief that most aerobic activities are similar, there are, in fact, major differences in aerobic activities performed at the same metabolic cost. Swimming and cycling, for example, are both non-weight bearing whereas running is not. Task characteristics such as the predictability of the sport environment (i.e., temporal-spatial certainty), probability of physical harm, and directness of competition seem to influence a sport preference (Berger, 1972, 1977). These three factors also might influence the potential psychological benefits of exercise. In highly predictable environments such as jogging and swimming, the exerciser is free to tune into his or her own thoughts and feelings. However, in temporally-spatially uncertain sport environments such as tennis and basketball, participants must focus their attention on a constantly changing environment. Exercisers in both types of sports may feel less anxious after physical exertion if the selected exercise mode is personalized. Swimmers might feel better because of the opportunity for internal dialogue permitted while swimming (Berger & Mackenzie, 1980). Tennis players might report less anxiety and depression after exercising as a result of forgetting everything except returning the ball. Of course, focusing exclusively on beating one's opponent might induce anxiety. Sport participants who do not choose an activity that is congruent with their needs may nor report psychological benefits.

It is conceivable that many aspects of the sport environment facilitate stress reduction. Because of the similarities between jogging and swimming, we decide to extend the focus of aerobic research by investigating the mood effects of swimming. Both swimming and jogging are aerobic, require little monitoring of the external environment, are rhythmical and repetitive in nature, and do not require vigilance as do other aerobic activities, such as racquet sports.

MOOD BENEFITS OF SWIMMING

Preliminary research results indicated that swimmers scored higher on anxiety than do other college students (Berger & Mashaback, 1980), and that their anxiety was related to mid-term swimming performance (Berger, 1979a). In a subsequent study, the Profile of Mood States (POMS) inventory (McNair, Lorr & Droppleman, 1971) was administered to four separate classes before and after 40 minutes of swimming near the end of a 14-week semester (Berger & Owen, 1983). The subjects represented two beginning and two intermediate swimming classes, as well as two classes of control subjects who did not exercise. As hypothesized the swimmers reported significant mood benefits on five of the six scales. They were significantly less tense ($p < .0002$), less depressed ($p < .0003$), less angry ($p < .001$), more vigorous ($p < .05$), and less confused ($p < .0002$) immediately following the swimming classes. Swimmers clearly "felt better" after swimming than they did before, and the psychological concomitants of swimming were very similar to those reported for running (Berger, 1984a; Morgan, 1979, Brown, Ramirez & Taub, 1978; Dienstier et al., 1981; Sachs & Buffone, 1984).

Swimmers' mood scores were compared with those of control students who attended lecture classes. The control group also enabled us to evaluate whether or not the college students who elected a swimming class differed from those who did not. This did not seem to be the case. No evidence was produced to indicate that the pre-class POMS scores of swimmers and controls differed, and this finding held for both males and females. However, the mean scores for both the swimmers and controls fell below the norms reported for the college students by the test authors (McNair et al., 1971). Since the swimmers were not anxious or depressed, and since their initial scores were below average, the improved affect argued against statistical regression as an explanation. It should be emphasized that the swimmers and controls were asked to respond to the instructional set of, "How do you feel right now?" as opposed to the set of "How you have been feeling during the past week including today" which was employed in the normative study (McNair et al., 1971, pp. 5, 19–20). In comparison with the non-exercising controls, swimmers reported significantly greater pre- to post-class changes on depression ($p < .05$), tension ($p < .06$), anger ($p < .002$), vigor ($p < .04$), and confusion ($p < .005$) (Berger & Owen, 1983).

Swimming requires an initial learning period in order for an individual to eventually exercise continuously for 20 to 30 minutes which has previously been suggested for mood enhancement (Berger, 1983/1984, 1984b; Dienstbier et al., 1981; Morgan, 1979). Therefore, it was hypothesized that the mood benefits of swimming would be greater for intermediate than for beginning swimmers. Since beginners and intermediates improved significantly on five of the six POMS scales this hypothesis was rejected. Testing occurred during the third month of bi-weekly instruction, and it is possible that beginners might not have reported mood changes earlier in the instructional process (Berger & Owen, 1983). A similar study was conducted during a five-week training session, but no changes in mood state were observed (Berger & Owen, 1986). However, this finding was probably due to numerous differences in experimental design rather than a failure to replicate. In view of subsequent data collected on the same swimmers, it seemed that the uncontrollably high air temperature of 106 °F which occurred on the day of testing occluded any mood benefits that might have occurred (Berger & Owen, in review).

STATE AND TRAIT ANXIETY

Analysis of swimmers' anxiety scores as measured by the State-Trait Anxiety Inventory (Spielberger, Gorsuch & Lushene, 1970) further supported the mood benefits of swimming (Berger & Own, in review). As hypothesized, swimmers reported significantly less state anxiety after swimming than before as measured on the first day of class, mid-semester, and at the end of the term. This was true both for swimmers in a 14-week Fall Term ($p < .00005$), as well as those in a 5-week Summer Term ($p < .00005$). The amount of anxiety reduction was comparable for beginners and intermediates as well as women and men.

Despite our expectation that a person might need to be a fairly proficient swimmer in order to realize any anxiety-reducing benefits, we found no evidence to support the skill-contingency hypothesis. Beginning and intermediate swimmers consistently reported mood benefits in these studies (Berger & Owen, 1983, in review). It is possible that the beginning swimmers may have been exercising strenuously even at the outset of the term. Moving in the shallow end of a pool, and practicing beginning skills, might require considerably more exertion for the neophyte than for the skilled swimmer. In other words, the beginners might have been exercising from their first day in the class at an intensity sufficient to produce improved mood states.

LONG–TERM EFFECTS

This research effort has not produced evidence of long-term benefits of swimming on anxiety. It appears that swimmers must return for additional swimming if they want to reduce their daily anxiety levels. In a recent investigation, we evaluated state anxiety before and after class on three occasions as well as trait anxiety on the first day of swimming and before and after the third day of testing (Berger & Owen, in review). Results indicated that short-term changes in state and trait anxiety following swimming did not persist at a long-term level.

An effort was also made to evaluate the possibility that swimmers who were high in somatic anxiety (Schwartz, Davidson & Goleman, 1978) would report greater reductions in state anxiety than would those with low somatic anxiety (Berger & Owen, in review). This hypothesis was not confirmed, and these results challenge the generalizability of the theory of anxiety proposed by Davidson and Schwartz (1976). This theory suggests the possibility of prescribing exercises as a means of reducing somatic anxiety, and cognitive approaches such as meditation for reducing psychic anxiety. Additional research is needed on this particular topic.

CONCLUSIONS

1. Swimmers are less anxious, depressed, angry, and more clear minded and vigorous after swimming than before, but the cause(s) for the mood enhancement is/are not clear.
2. These changes seem to be short-term rather than long-term.
3. Women and men report similar mood benefits.
4. Both beginning and intermediate swimmers report stress reducing benefits.

14

EXERCISE IN THE PREVENTION AND TREATMENT OF DEPRESSION

Wesley E. Sime

INTRODUCTION

The impact of regular physical activity of a vigorous nature upon psychological mood states is quite remarkable. It is remarkable because it seems to foster great expression of enthusiasm for some, and by contrast, for others it is a most abhorent, distasteful almost painful experience. It is likely that past experience with social reinforcement, secondary gain, and personal satisfaction being associated with sport, manual labor or recreation (or the lack of such an association) parameter probably accounts for the disparity in personal feelings about exercise.

Most health scientists agree that exercise has a positive effect upon physical well-being and upon specific physiological variables associated with health and wellness. (e.g., heart rate, blood pressure). A similar convincing body of evidence is, as yet, lacking regarding the beneficent effect of exercise upon mental well-being. As background perspective for this chapter, it should be noted that as recently as two decades ago, evidence supporting the physiological benefits of exercise was equally as week, poorly controlled, biased and empirical as the absence of compelling evidence on the psychological benefits now under scrutiny. I intend to show some parallels between the two and point in a direction with some prospect for more unanimous agreement on the issues.

At the outset, let me acknowledge the fact that the literature regarding exercise and mental health is voluminous but lacking sound, reliable research design methods (Folkins & Sime, 1981; Morgan, 1984). Over 1100 articles were located in one review (Hughes, 1984) but only 14 of these met the criteria for adequate experimental controls. I am impressed by the fact that there seems to be far too many articles critiquing the literature on exercise/depression and far too few articles reporting actual work with clinically depressed patients utilizing vigorous exercise (Hughes, 1984; Weinstein & Meyers, 1983; Ledwidge, 1980; Browman, 1981; Buffone, 1984; Berger, 1984a). Thus, I submit to you herein, that we will *not* see the interest nor the funding to support it until the empirical and clinical efficacy becomes considerably stronger. This efficacy will not necessarily be achieved with very large populations, but perhaps will be aided by a non-traditional pioneering approach. With that in mind, I am going to trace the history of my personal involvement with this research question.

Trained as an exercise physiologist specializing in cardiac rehabilitation, I had a long history of frustration with the lack of supportive research data on the benefits of exercise (Sime, Whipple, Stamler, & Berkson, 1978). As that volume of evidence began to accumulate (Berkson, Whipple, MacIntyre, Sime & Stamler, 1969; Sime, 1971; Holloszy, 1983; Shephard, Corey & Kavanaugh, 1981), I gradually changed emphasis toward psychophysiology and the potential for reducing muscle tension both with exercise (Sime, 1978; 1981) and with instrumentation-based biofeedback and relaxation (Sime & DeGood, 1977a; Sime & DeGood, 1977b). The growing interest in the latter, together with a logical, analytical approach to emotional stress testing (Sime, Buell, Eliot, 1980a; Sime, Buell, Eliot, 1980b) dominated my concern for some time with regards to emotional stress testing. Our research efforts grew rapidly with an NIMH grant that allowed us to focus upon occupational stress variables, as well as various coping techniques of the average adult employee. Therein lies the basis for Study I. At the same time, however, I was drawn closer to psychological and clinical issues with studies in psychophysiology. A doctoral candidate in psychology sought my assistance in testing the anti-depressant effects of exercise. The results of the effort and the follow-up served as the basis for Study II reported herein.

My personal initiative in this area came forth somewhat paradoxically during the past year. I had been gradually evolving away from the science of physical activity toward biofeedback and stress management. In the process, I became a referral source for psychologists and psychiatrists who had moderately depressed patients that were not candidates for anti-depressant drug therapy or who were not responding to psychotherapy. Having assurance that all medical and psychological needs were being met with these patients, I was willing to accept them in a stress management program. Very quickly, I too, discovered that a more potent and multi-faceted approach was necessary with these patients. Drawing upon personal experiences and the anecdotal experience of others (Sime, 1979; Greist, Kline, Eischens, Faris, Gorman & Morgan, 1979; Kostrubala, 1981; Kostrubala, 1984), I began systematically introducing an exercise therapy program. Much to my surprise I realized that, in a way, I had come full circle from an exercise physiology perspective through psychophysiology and back again to exercise therapy. Therein lies the background for the third study to be reported in this chapter.

STUDY I

Approximately 700 employees were recruited for participation in an occupational stress study. Numerous physiological, behavioral and psychological variables were obtained in assessing both the employer and the employee. Some of these results have been reported (Sime, Mayes, Witte, Ganston, & Tharp, 1985). In general, the results indicate that personal strain and organizational performance can be influenced by the stress imposed by the job environment or by the perception thereof by the employee.

The data from this study, which bears impact upon the mental health question, is focused upon the leisure time activity reports of the employee. Table 1 shows the leisure time variables remaining in the regression equation with depression as a dependent variable. It is apparent that the report of depression is clearly associated in a positive direction ($P < .001$) with the frequency of recreational drug usage (e.g., marijuana), and negatively ($P < 0.05$) with reading and sport activity. While reading and sport might have similar diversionary qualities, it is interesting to note that the amount of television viewing is proportional by association, with the level of depression. It is possible that just watching the news on TV can be a depressing experience for some individuals.

Table 1 also shows the leisure variables remaining in the regression equation with anxiety as the dependent variable. Again, reading was associated with lower levels of anxiety ($p < 0.01$), while TV ($p < 0.05$) and music ($p < 0.05$)

TABLE 1   Leisure activity variables remaining in regression equations with depression and anxiety as the dependent variables. (N = 412).

Activity variables	Beta	r
Depression		
Drug use (recreational)	0.167***	0.177
Reading (books, magazines)	—0.104*	—0.122
Sport (outdoor recreation basketball, softball, etc.)	—0.100*	—0.097
Television (watching)	0.088+	0.078
Multiple R	0.242	
R Square	0.059	
Anxiety		
Music (listening)	0.825*	0.049
Yoga (stretching)	—0.049	—0.062
Television (watching)	0.077*	0.065
Smoking	0.052	0.063
Reading (books, magazines)	—0.102**	—0.089
Sport (outdoor recreation basketball, softball, etc.)	—0.072+	—0.066
Jogging	0.001	0.037
Multiple R	0.17	
R Square	0.029	

+p $\leq$ 0.10
*p $\leq$ 0.05
**p $\leq$ 0.01
***p $\leq$ 0.001

were *positively* associated with anxiety levels. Both jogging and yoga were reported by so few participants (predominantly blue collar) that they would not be likely to enter into the equation. It would appear as though anxiety and depression share some of the same concordant characteristics in this population. The bivariate correlation between anxiety and depression was r = 0.81, thus accounting for the joint association between the two.

These descriptive data suggest that the level of anxiety and depression in a free living-working, non-clinical population is associated with the leisure behavior therein. More specifically, watching TV and recreational drug usage are associated with higher levels of depression, while reading and sport (seemingly "quality" leisure activities) are associated with less depression in this population. Similarly, reading and sport are associated with less depression while watching TV and listening to music (rock and country music, not classical) are associated with higher levels of depression. Given these cross-sectional results, it would seem appropriate to embark upon intervention research, particularly with depression. This investigation served as the background for studies two and three.

STUDY II

Vigorous exercise is a functional self-regulatory activity that enhances physiological and homeostasis. It has been described as a very potent cathartic agent emotionally as well as physically. Theories regarding the physiological mechanism to account for the anti-depressant effect of exercise include:

1. The apparent increase in blood flow and oxygenation to the central nervous system (Friedlander, 1981).
2. Popular opinion that increased blood endorphin levels reduce pain and elevate mood though recent evidence contradicts this hypothesis (Flynn, Mitchell and Goldfarb, 1985), and controversy exists whether endorphin levels could influence mood based upon naloxone blocking studies (Markoff, Ryan, & Young, 1982).
3. Enhanced aminergic synaptic transmission (Ransford, 1982).
4. The increase in urine norepinephrine levels (Dienstbier, 1981; Dienstbier, 1984) which may be indicative of other metabolic changes involving catecholamines in the mood swings.

Previous research suggests that the most effective exercise prescription for an anti-depressant effect is about the same as that recommended for cardiovascular benefits. A slow gradual progression of exercise up to 3–5 times per week, at 70–85% of maximum aerobic capacity for about 20–60 minutes is recommended (Eischens & Greist, 1984; Berger, 1984b). Further, it is suggested that: 1) A routine be established; 2) Enjoyment and self-mastery be encouraged with the possibility that enhanced self-esteem will result; and 3)

Additional self-satisfaction be achieved by keeping a log of accumulated progress, by establishing a behavioral contract to achieve a specific goal, and by the psychodynamics involved in exercising together in a group. These factors were incorporated into the study described next.

A multiple baseline study with cross-sectional times eries analyses was used on a population of 15 moderately depressed subjects (Sime & Sanstead, 1985). They ranged in age from 26–53 years and all were employed, though 8 worked only part-time. Five were divorced, 7 were married and 3 were single. Each subject served as their own control in this multiple baseline across-subjects-design wherein multiple measures of depression were obtained over several weeks of screening and a 2 week baseline which preceded the 10 week exercise program. The Beck Depression Inventory, the Profile of Mood States and a Daily Mood Scale were used to assess depression levels periodically throughout this study. Three of the fifteen subjects had to drop out early for logistical reasons (accident, illness and relocation). To account for possible socialization effects and the possible effects due to the instructor, an extra baseline (placebo exercise consisting of stretching and calisthenics [non-aerobics]) was provided for 2 weeks prior to the actual aerobic treatment program. No change in depression levels were observed following the placebo exercise, thus baseline data in Table 2 is an average of pre-training and placebo. The aerobic exercise program was instituted 4 times/week at a gradually increasing level with instructor support both in the group and individually. A progressive increase in exercise tolerance occurred throughout the study although fitness evaluations on a bicycle ergometer did not show a significant increase in cardiovascular fitness, perhaps due to the problem of cross specificity of training and testing (i.e., walk/run training versus bicycle testing). In spite of this failure to show fitness level increases, there was a significant decrease in Beck Depression Scores, particularly at 6-month follow-up (Table 2). Of the original 15 subjects, 13 were located for interview, and 2 were lost to follow-up immediately due to relocation. Ten of the 13 reported depression levels the same or lower than at the finish of the exercise program. Four of the 13 reported continuing in the running program at the same frequency/intensity/duration or greater and another 5 reported equivalent exercise in the form of aerobics, minim-tramp, stationary bicycle or hard physical labor (occupational). The 3 who were more depressed at follow-up had no reported exercise

TABLE 2   Beck depression at baseline, following exercise at six- and twenty-one month follow-up

Baseline	Exercise	6-month Follow-up	21-month Follow-up
$\overline{X}$ = 14.2	9.4*	9.2*	8.3*
SE = 1.0	1.0	1.0	2.0

*Significantly different from baseline (p < .01).

habits and the other subject who showed increased mood, attributed it to a change from running to yoga stretching, which served her personal needs much better. All of the 10 subjects who showed increased mood, reported that their participation in the original exercise program had increased their awareness of fitness benefits (self-esteem, self-mastery) regardless of whether they continued to jog or shifted to another form of exercise at follow-up.

This multiple baseline, time-series study tends to support the hypothe-sized beneficial effect (psychological) of vigorous exercise. The outcome of this long-term follow-up, even in a quasi-experimental time-series study, is rare and presumably nonexistant by perusal of previous reviews (Folkins & Sime, 1981; Morgan, 1984; Hughes, 1984; Berger, 1984; Weinstein & Meyers, 1983).

STUDY III

Selected Case Study

J. D. was a 38-year-old divorced male with a compulsive, perfectionistic personality and with a two year history of severe anxiety and depression follow-ing an anxiety attack that included severe non-cardiac chest pain. There was no organic cause for pain. A psychiatrist prescribed Halcion (benzodiazopene tran-quilizer) and Surmontal (mild sedative, anti-depressant) and kept increasing dosage in spite of side effects and minimal symptom relief until the patient became psychologically addicted. Following shock treatment and 30 days in a drug withdrawal center, the patient returned to work and was referred for stress management.

Intervention

With assurance that his psychological and medical needs were being met, this therapist embarked upon intervention of combined biofeedback and exer-cise therapy. Chest paint symptoms reported earlier were traced to myositis in the pectoralis muscles of the chest. Biofeedback, myotherapy and stretching exercises were effective in relieving the chest pain, but the anxiety/depression mood swings persisted. A program of gradually increasing walk/jog exercises was instituted. It should be noted here that a recommendation from a counselor to exercise was not sufficient. While most psychiatrist verbalize the benefits of exercise (Byrd, 1963), very few actually incorporate it into therapy. In reality, most depressed patients can't "get it together" to start an exercise program of their own initiative. In the present case study, the patient was too anxious and fearful to join a group exercise program and was too depressed to start exercis-ing on his own. Thus it was necessary to personally conduct the exercise ther-apy. Serendipitously, the cathartic effects of physical exertion carried over into the psychological catharsis. More rational and spontaneous expression were observed in the midst of the exercise sessions as this information was systemati-cally transmitted to the referring psychiatrist and psychologist. It would, of course, be preferable to have the counseling therapist also conduct the exercise therapy, but very few will do it (Kostrubala, 1984).

Results

Figure 1 shows the temporal association between mood state (depression) and exercise habits over a 5 week period preceded by an 8 week baseline. In perusing the temporal alignment of occasions/intensity of exercise with mood state (depression) it would appear as though the acute effects are fairly dramatic. It should also be noted that these anti-depressant effects are transient and not persistent for more than 12–26 hours following each bout. That would appear to corroborate the theory that aminergic synaptic transmission is enhanced immediately following an acute bout of exercise (Ransford, 1982). This patient continues to have periodic mood swings and psychological therapy aimed at cognitive restructuring, but the exercise remains the most potent, acute anti-depressant agent.

Similar case study results (with less severe depression problems and thus less dramatic results) have been observed by this therapist. Without discussing each in detail, I can report that it is the most frustrating work I have ever encountered, yet it can also be the most rewarding. Resistance to therapy and reluctancy to acknowledge progressive improvement is, of course, quite prevalent. At times, I think the depression becomes a communicator disease which is temporarily passed on to the therapist, making the exercise sessions even more crucial. I spite of these difficulties there is great satisfaction in collaborating in a therapeutic process which averts self-destructive tendencies and may even prevent suicide.

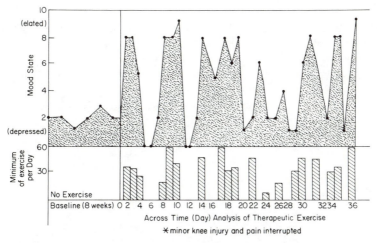

FIGURE 1   Mood state (depression) plotted in temporal comparison with exercise (walk/run) in minutes/day for one severely anxious/depressed suicidal patient.

SUMMARY

Multiple approaches have been utilized in describing the relationship between exercise and depression. A descriptive study with a large population occupational stress focus was useful in demonstrating an apparent associative (non-causal) link between leisure activity (sport) and anxiety/depression. Though another quality, diversion (reading) was more significant, the value of exercise (sport) was apparent.

Two additional quasi-experimental studies were presented. In the first, a single case design, multiple baseline, time series study with 15 subjects showed that depression levels were decreased with vigorous exercise and these effects were maintained (and perhaps enhanced) over a 21 month follow-up. The long-term follow-up and the use of a placebo-exercise treatment (which had no impact) is definitely unique in studies of this nature. The last study in this series is very narrowly focused upon one very severely depressed patient. The temporal association between acute bouts of exercise and mood state (depression) is quite dramatic and would seem to plan further conviction among the optimistic empiricists who support the role of exercise in the prevention and treatment of depression.

While the bulk of literature in this area lacks the necessary experimental control to document a causal role for exercise as an anti-depressant agent, there is more than sufficient suggestive data to foster support for a large scale clinical trial in this area (Blumenthal, Williams, Needels, & Wallace, 1982). Realistically, however, that will not take place, until the popular trend (critically reviewing the literature) is shifted to more efficacious studies (clinically and empirically) that employ unique and innovative therapeutic approaches.

IV

APPLICATIONS AND FUTURE DIRECTIONS

15

SUMMARY

William P. Morgan and Stephen E. Goldston

INTRODUCTION

Bloom (1985) has reported that during the course of any given year 15 percent of the American population suffer from various emotional disorders. It has also been estimated that almost 7 million of these 32 million individuals "receive no care of any kind (p. 3)." These statistics are significant for a number of reasons. First, the 15% figure represents a significant increase over the 10% (1 out of 10) figure that has historically been cited in estimating the number of Americans with emotional or psychiatric disorders at any given point in time. In other words, even though the capacity of our mental health delivery system to provide care has expanded, the incidence of health problems has increased (Bloom, 1985).

The only sensible approach to the control of today's major health problems will occur through *prevention*, not *treatment*. A number of comprehensive volumes dealing with prevention of stress-related psychiatric disorders have been published in recent years (Albee & Joffee, 1977; Bloom, 1985; Goldman & Goldston, 1985). There is also compelling evidence that prevention involves the preferred approach to other major health problems such as cardiovascular disease (Lenfant & Schweizer, 1985). Also, disease prevention and health promotion have become central concerns in recent policy efforts at the federal level (McGinnis, 1985).

The extent to which habitual physical activity can play a role in the primary and secondary prevention of emotional disorders has been considered in this volume. An effort has been made to elucidate *that which we know* about the relationship at present, as well as *that which we should strive to know* in the future. The consensus statements which follow are based upon "the-state-of-the-art" of present knowledge.

CONSENSUS STATEMENTS

Consensus Statements Relating To What We Know: Research Evidence

Exercise and Mental Health:

1. Physical fitness is positively associated with mental health and well-being.
2. Exercise is associated with the reduction of stress emotions such as state anxiety.
3. Anxiety and depression are common symptoms of failure to cope with mental stress, and exercise has been associated with a decreased level of mild to moderate depression and anxiety.
4. Longterm exercise is usually associated with reductions in traits such as neuroticism and anxiety.
5. Severe depression usually requires professional treatment which may include medication, electroconvulsive therapy, and/or psychotherapy, with exercise as an adjunct.
6. Appropriate exercise results in reductions in various stress indices such as neuromuscular tension, resting heart rate, and some stress hormones.
7. Current clinical opinion holds that exercise has beneficial emotional effects across all ages and in both sexes.
8. Physically healthy people who require psychotropic medication may safely exercise when exercise and medications are titrated under close medical supervision.

Programmatic Issues:

1. We know how to conceptualize (define) primary and secondary prevention programs in which exercise can be a fundamental component.
2. We know how to develop a comprehensive information system involving exercise and mental health.
3. An improvement in psychological status, including an enhanced ability to cope with mental stress, frequently accompanies exercise programs that produce an increase in aerobic capacity. Programs with different characteristics (e.g., exercise type, intensity, amount or frequency) may also provide similar benefits, but they have not been adequately tested.
4. Maintenance of an active lifestyle usually requires a concerted, sustained effort in which the individual remains attentive to making exercise a regular part of living.

5. Use of exercise to treat behavioral-emotional disorders associated with stress should be preceded by a thorough assessment of each individual's medical-behavioral-emotional-social-environmental functioning.
6. Maintenance of a regular exercise program is a critical aspect of exercise as a means of coping with mental stress.
7. Adherence rates in exercise programs vary widely from high to low, but typically, 50% of participants will drop out within three to six months.
8. Both programmatic features and personal characteristics are associated with exercise adherence.
9. Many of those persons most likely to benefit from regular exercise are not likely to begin or continue an exercise program unless attention is paid to individual reinforcement factors.
10. Several health risk behaviors (e.g., smoking, overweight) are associated with dropping out of exercise programs, and these factors are difficult, but not impossible, to change.

Consensus Statements Relating To What We Need To Know: Research Needs

Exercise and Mental Health:

1. Moderate exercise has been found to be superior to meprobamate in its immediate effect upon neuromuscular tension in older adults. Additional studies are needed to compare exercise with (newer) benzodiazepine anxiolytics.
2. What is the role of exercise in the primary prevention of mental and physical disorders?
3. What is the effect of exercise on the rehabilitation of individuals with various physical and mental disorders?
4. What are the mechanisms (e.g., biological, cognitive, psychological, social) that mediate the beneficial effects of exercise on reactions to mental stress?
5. What are the effects of exercise on stress reactions for persons differing in personality traits, age, sex, and socio-cultural (SES) backgrounds?
6. What is the optimal mode, intensity, duration, and frequency of exercise required to produce more effective responses to mental stress?
7. What is the effect of exercise in comparison to, and in combination with, other approaches to stress reduction such as drug therapy, psychotherapy and other stress management programs?
8. Research leading to knowledge about the role of exercise in the prevention and treatment of depression is needed.

9. What are the effects of exercise on the mental health of children?
10. What are the effects of exercise on the following disorders: substance abuse, schizophrenia, personality disorders (esp. antisocial and borderline), sleep disorders, eating disorders, psychosexual disorders, psychosomatic disorders, bipolar disorders, and severe unipolar depression?
11. Can exercise increase the effectiveness of psychotropic medications?
12. Can exercise reduce the need for, or side-effects of, psychotropic medications?
13. What are the effects of exercise on cognitive processes including memory, body image and self-concept?
14. What is the potential role of exercise in the management of mental stress in physical disorders such as cancer, diabetes, renal failure and arthritis?
15. What are the mechanisms underlying exercise effects? For example, what is the role of rhythmicity, proprioception, temperature changes, biogenic amines, endorphins, time-out, self-efficacy/mastery, and other life style factors (e.g., smoking, nutrition, sleep, work, substance use)?

Programmatic Issues:

1. What are the cost-benefits of various approaches designed to prevent sedentary living? For example, how effective are methods designed to modify the environment and attempts to increase "life-style" exercising (e.g., walking up stairs more, parking further from shopping centers and work, etc.)?
2. Why and when do sedentary life-styles develop?
3. Which prevention strategies apply best to which target populations?
4. How can one assess (reliably and validly) sedentary life-styles?
5. Who will benefit most from existing programmatic approaches or from approaches designed to increase routine or life-style activity?
6. Need exists to evaluate the nature of various change agents (e.g., family, media, community, programmatic).
7. Need exists to examine the interactions of other health related behaviors in facilitating exercise behavior and vice versa.
8. What reinforces exercise behaviors among the habitually active?
9. Why do people discontinue exercise programs?
10. What are the preferred types, intensity, frequency, and duration of exercise programs needed to insure adherence?
11. More reliable and valid measures of exercise adherence are needed.
12. How do individuals start and maintain exercise programs on their own initiative, and what are the characteristics of these people?
13. The dose-response relationship between exercise intensity and amount with various psychological benefits needs to be defined.

14. Due to the low participation rates for middle-aged and older Americans with higher intensity programs, there is a need to investigate alternative approaches to increasing exercise among these groups.

15. Need exists to provide a framework within which a comprehensive bibliographic data base can be further developed and maintained to address concerns about exercise and its effects on mental health.

BIBLIOGRAPHY: A RETRIEVAL SYSTEM FOR EXERCISE AND MENTAL HEALTH

Michael L. Sachs

INTRODUCTION

Information management is an important component of any scientific field. The wealth of publications and presentations in each field provides a vast quantity of information that is of potential use to investigators and practitioners. Critical areas of information management include information storage, retrieval, and dissemination. The bibliography contained in this chapter relates primarily to information retrieval and dissemination; a discussion of its development follows.

BIBLIOGRAPHIC DATA BASES

Bibliographic data bases have been in existence for a number of years. These data bases include thousands of references from books, journals, presentations at conferences, and other sources. Through the use of selected "keys" (e.g., type of article, year of publication, journal name) and key words (e.g., anxiety, depression, exercise), the investigator and practitioner can locate articles dealing with specific topics of interest. Hundreds of on-line data bases are accessible through government, college, university, and municipal libraries. Indeed, the oldest computer data-base dictionary, *Computer-readable Data Bases: A Directory and Data Source Book,* is 1500 pages thick and growing (Turner, 1983). Some of the more well-known data base services offered include Psychological Abstracts, Dialog Information Services, and the Medical Literature Analysis and Retrieval System (MEDLARS). These on-line systems can be accessed directly by a librarian and, working with the user, a data-base search can be performed in a cost- and time-efficient manner.

INFORMATION RETRIEVAL

The data bases noted above represent the storage of information, so that a readily accessible record of information can be easily *searched.* Of particular interest, of course, is the *retrieval* of this information. The user has several choices in his/her pursuit of bibliographic information (references dealing with a topic of interest). The first is to search through one of the commercially available on-line data bases for relevant references. This is a systematic and time-efficient method, but can be costly if the time required for searching is extensive and the number of references obtained is large.

Depending on the user's needs, there are various information retrieval systems that have already been developed for professionals in the exercise and sport sciences. In particular, a number of indexes are available which regularly review the major publications, books, and other sources for references of interest. These and other sources have been reviewed by Crase and Sachs (1980). Some of these sources are no longer in existence (e.g., Runner's Index), but most are still available.

The final choice or option is a less systematic search by the researcher through various journals and other publications on a regular or irregular basis in an effort to remain current. This type of search may reveal numerous articles of interest, but can also result in some references being missed.

BIBLIOGRAPHY ON PSYCHOLOGICAL CONSIDERATIONS IN EXERCISE

The approach used in developing the bibliography on psychological considerations in exercise has been, in a sense, both systematic and unsystematic. The foundation for the bibliography was laid in 1976 with a thesis by Sharon Burgess (Burgess, 1976) at Florida State University, and the author subsequently added references primarily through regular reviews of various sources.

1. *Current Contents* (Social & Behavioral Sciences; Clinical Practice) for relevant articles, using key words such as exercise, sports, and therapy.
2. New issues of journals that were most likely to contain relevant articles.
3. *Dissertation Abstracts International.*
4. Conference proceedings (such as those of the North American Society for the Psychology of Sport and Physical Activity, and the American College of Sports Medicine).
5. Reference lists of published articles or copies of presented papers for articles that had not been previously noted.

Although this approach was relatively systematic, a "thoroughly" systematic search would have included regular searches of on-line data bases. The above methods have provided, though, a reasonably comprehensive search of the available sources. It is certainly possible that one will miss an occasional article, but generally "someone will find it" and it will appear in a published article at some point in the future. Careful checks of all likely sources suggest that almost all articles of any importance will be found in this manner. Additionally, the methods noted above ensure that one will have as one's companion the "Prince of Serendip," and one may find references on other subjects that are of interest and value for other research efforts by one's self, colleagues, and students.

The methods cited are the same ones that can be used to develop any bibliography, either building upon the existing ones involving "psychological considerations," or dealing with another area entirely. Most investigators have an 'informal' listing of relevant references in a number of existing publications, and once these are compiled, the beginnings of a useful and comprehensive bibliography in a specific area of interest exists.

The following bibliography is not comprehensive since it has been restricted to those references cited by the authors of the chapters in the present volume. It can be used to check on these references, or the user might wish to simply browse through the listing in search of articles of potential interest.

BIBLIOGRAPHY

Ajzen, I., & Fishbein, M. (1977). Attitude-behavior relations: A theoretical analysis and review of empirical research. *Psychological Bulletin, 84,* 888–918.

Akiskal, H. S., & McKinney, W. T. (1975). Overview of recent research in depression: Integration of ten conceptual models into a comprehensive clinical frame. *Archives of General Psychiatry, 32,* 285–305.

Aksnes, E. G. (1977). Beta-blokker: Farlig for skilopere? Tidsskrift for den Norske Laegeforening, *12,* 576.

Albee, G. W., & Joffee, J. M. (Eds.). (1977). *The primary prevention of psychopathology: The issues.* Hanover, NH: University Press of New England.

Allen, L. D., & Iwata, B. A. (1980). Reinforcing exercise maintenance using high-rate activities. *Behavior Modification, 4,* 337–354.

American College of Sports Medicine (1978, July). Position statement on the recommended quantity and quality of exercise for developing and maintaining fitness in healthy adults. *Sports Medicine Bulletin, 13(1),* 3–4.

American Medical Association. (1983, November 7). Personal health care. *Newsweek* (advertising supplement).

American Psychiatric Association. (1980). Diagnostic and statistical manual of mental disorders (3rd ed.). Washington, DC: Author.

American Running and Fitness Association. (1981). Statistical report. Washington, DC: Author.

Andersen, S. D., Bye, P. T. P., Perry, C. P., Hamor, G. P., Theobald, G., & Nyberg, G. (1979). Limitation of work performance in normal adult males in the presence of beta-adrenergic blocade. *Australian New Zealand Journal of Medicine, 9,* 515–520.

Andrew, G. M., Oldridge, N. B., Parker, J. O., Cunningham, D. A., Rechnitzer, P. A., Jones, N. L., Buck, C., Kavanagh, T., Shephard, R. J., Sutton, J. R., & McDonald, W. (1981). Reasons for dropout from exercise programs in postcoronary patients. *Medicine and Science in Sports and Exercise, 13(3),* 164–168.

Andrew, G. M., & Parker, J. O. (1979). Factors related to dropout of post myocardial infarction patients from exercise programs. *Medicine and Science in Sports and Exercise, 11*, 376–378.

Angel, R. W., & Hofmann, W. W. (1963). The H reflex in normal, spastic and rigid subjects. *Archives of Neurology, 8*, 591–596.

Asberg, M., Perris, C., Schalling, D., & Sedvall, G. (1978). The CPRS-development and applications of a psychiatric rating scale. *Acta Psychiatrica Scandinavica, 271* (Suppl.), 1–27.

Astrand, P. O., & Rodahl, K. (1977). *Textbook of work physiology.* New York: McGraw-Hill.

Badenhop, D. T., Cleary, P. A., Schall, S. F., Fox, E. L., & Bartels, R. (1983). Physiologic adjustments to higher or lower intensity exercise in elders. *Medicine and Science in Sports and Exercise, 15*, 496–502.

Baekeland, F. (1970). Exercise deprivation: Sleep and psychological reactions. *Archives of General Psychiatry, 22*, 365–369.

Bahrke, M. S., & Morgan, W. P. (1978). Anxiety reduction following exercise and meditation. *Cognitive Therapy and Research, 2*, 323–333.

Baile, W. F., & Engel, B. T. (1979). A behavioral strategy for promoting treatment compliance following myocardial infarction. In C. M. Franck & G. T. Wilson (Eds.), *Annual Review of Behavior Therapy* (Vol. 7). New York: Brunner/Mazel.

Ballantyne, D., Clark, A., Dyker, G. S., Gillis, C. R., Hawthorne, V. M., Henry, D. A., Hole, D. S., Murdoch, R. M., Semple, T., & Stewart, G. M. (1978, July). Prescribing exercise for the healthy: Assessment of compliance and effects of plasma lipids and lipoproteins. *Health Bulletin, 36*, 169–176.

Balog, L. F. (1983). The effects of exercise on muscle tension and subsequent muscle relaxation training. *Research Quarterly, 54*, 119–125.

Balshan, I. D. (1962). Muscle tension and personality in women. *Archives of General Psychiatry, 7*, 436–448.

Baranowski, T., Dworkin, R. J., Cieslikk, C. J., Hooks, P., Clearman, D., Ray, L., Dunn, J., & Nader, P. (1984). Reliability and validity of self-report of aerobic activity: Family health project. *Research Quarterly for Exercise and Sport, 55*, 309–317.

Baun, W. B. (1984, May). *Exercise adherence: An update and critique.* Paper presented at the annual meeting of the American College of Sports Medicine, San Diego, CA.

Bayles, C., Laporte, R., Petrini, A., Cauley, J., Slemenda, C., & Sandler, R. B. (1984). A comparison of compliers and non-compliers in a randomized exercise trail of 229 post-menopausal women (Abstract). *Medicine and Science in Sports and Exercise, 16*, 115.

Beary, J. F., & Benson, H. (1974). A simple psychophysiologic technique which elicits the hypometabolic changes of the relaxation response. *Psychosomatic Medicine, 31*, 115–120.

Beck, A. T., Rush, A. J., Shaw, B. F., & Emery, G. (1979). *Cognitive therapy of depression.* New York: Guilford Press.

Becker, M. H. (1974). The health belief model and personal health behavior. *Health Education Monographs, 2*, 326.

Belloc, N. B., & Breslow, L. (1972). Relationship of health status and health practices. *Preventive Medicine, 1,* 409-421.

Benfari, R. C., Eaker, E., & Stoll, J. G. (1981). Behavioral interventions and compliance to treatment regimes. *Annual Review of Public Health, 2,* 431-471.

Berger, B. G. (1972). Relationships between the environmental factors or temporal-spatial uncertainty, probability of physical harm, and nature of competition and selected personality characteristics of athletes. *Dissertation Abstracts International, 33,* 1014A. (University Microfilms No. 72-23689, 373)

Berger, B. G. (1977). Effect of uncertainty, physical harm, and competition upon selected personality characteristics of athletes. *International Journal of Sport Psychology, 8,* 198-209.

Berger, B. G. (1979a, June). *Influence of state and trait anxiety upon learning of beginning and intermediate swimmers.* Paper presented at the International Congress of Physical Education, Trois-Rivieres, Quebec, Canada.

Berger, B. G. (1979b). The meaning of regular jogging: A phenomenological approach. In R. H. Cox (Ed.), *American Alliance for Health, Physical Education and Recreation Research Consortium Papers:* Health, fitness, recreation, and dance, (Vol. 2, Book 2). Washington, DC: Author.

Berger, B. G. (1982). Facts and fancy: Mood alteration through exercise. *Journal of Physical Education, Recreation, and Dance, 53*(9), 47-48.

Berger, B. G. (1983/1984). Stress reduction through exercise: The mind-body connection. *Motor Skills: Theory into Practice, 7*(2), 31-46.

Berger, B. G. (1984a). Running away from anxiety and depression: A female as well as male race. In M. L. Sachs & G. W. Buffone (Eds.), *Running as therapy: An integrated approach.* Lincoln, NE: University of Nebraska Press.

Berger, B. G. (1984b). Running strategies for women and men. In M. L. Sachs & G. W. Buffone (Eds.), *Running as therapy: An integrated approach.* Lincoln, NE: University of Nebraska Press.

Berger, B. G. (1984c). Running toward psychological well-being: Special considerations for the female client. In M. L. Sachs & G. W. Buffone (Eds.), *Running as therapy: An integrated approach.* Lincoln, NE: University of Nebraska Press.

Berger, B. G. (1986). Use of jogging and swimming as stress reduction techniques. In J. H. Humphrey (Ed.), *Human Stress: Current selected research in human stress* (Vol. 1). (pp. 169-190). New York: AMS Press.

Berger, B. G., & Mackenzie, M. M. (1980). A case study of a woman jogger: A psychodynamic analysis. *Journal of Sport Behavior, 3,* 3-16.

Berger, B. G., & Mushabac, L. (1978). Effect of swimming ability and sex on state and trait anxiety of students in college swimming classes. In G. C. Roberts & K. M. Newell (Eds.), *Psychology of motor behavior and sport.* (pp. 26-35), Champaign, IL: Human Kinetics Publishers.

Berger, B. G., & Owen, D. R. (1983). Mood alteration with swimming—swimmers really do "feel better." *Psychosomatic Medicine, 45*(5), 425-433.

Berger, B. G., & Owen, D. R. (1986). Mood alteration with swimming: A re-examination. In J. H. Humphrey & L. Vander Velden (Eds.), *Psychology and sociology of sport: Current selected research,* (Vol. 1, pp. 97-114). New York: AMS Press.

Berger, B. G., & Owen, D. R. (in review). *Anxiety reduction with swimming*. Manuscript submitted for publication. (a)

Berger, B. G., & Owen, D. R. (in review). *Mood alteration with swimming: A re-examination*. Manuscript submitted for publication. (b)

Berger, R. A., & Littlefield, D. H. (1969). Comparison between football athletes and non-athletes on personality. *Research Quarterly, 40,* 663.

Berkson, D., Whipple, I. P., MacIntyre, W., Sime, W., & Stamler, J. (1969). Results of short-duration, high-intensity ergometric exercise, *Circulation, 45* (Suppl. III), 39–40.

Bewsher, P. D. (1967). Propanolol, blood-sugar, and exercise. *Lancet,* 104.

Blair, S. N. (1982). Exercise and coronary heart disease. *Behavioral Medicine Update, 4,* 13–16.

Blair, S. N., Falls, H. R., & Pate, R. R. (1983, April). A new physical fitness. *The Physician and Sportsmedicine, 11,* 81–87, 94–95.

Blair, S. N., Jacobs, D. R., & Powell, K. E. (1985). Relationships between exercise or physical activity and other health behaviors. *Public Health Reports, 100*(2), 172–180.

Blair, S. N., Haskell, W. L., Ho, P., Paffenbarger, R. S., Vranizan, K. M., Farquhar, J. W., & Wood, P. D. (1985). Assessment of habitual physical activity by a seven-day recall in a community survey and controlled experiments. *American Journal of Epidemiology, 122,* 794–804.

Bloom, B. L. (1984). *Community mental health: A general introduction* (2nd ed.). Belmont, CA: Brooks/Cole.

Bloom, B. L. (1985a). Focal issues in the prevention of mental disorders. In H. H. Goldman, & S. E. Goldston (Eds.), *Preventing stress-related psychiatric disorders* (DHHS Publication No. ADM 85-1366). Washington, DC: U.S. Government Printing Office.

Bloom, B. L. (1985b). *Stressful life event theory and research: Implications for primary prevention* (DHHS Publication No. ADM 85-1385). Washington, DC: U.S. Government Printing Office.

Blue, F. R. (1979). Aerobic running as a treatment for moderate depression. *Perceptual and Motor Skills, 48,* 228.

Blumenthal, J. A., Schocken, D. D., Needles, T. L., & Hindle, P. (1982). Psychological and physiological effects of physical conditioning on the elderly. *Journal of Psychosomatic Research, 26,* 505–510.

Blumenthal, J. A., Williams, R., Needels, G., & Wallace, A. (1982). Psychological changes accompany aerobic exercise in healthy middle-aged adults. *Psychosomatic Medicine, 44,* 529–536.

Blumenthal, J. A., Williams, R. S., Wallace, A. G., Williams, R. B., & Needles, T. L. (1982). Physiological and psychological variables predict compliance to prescribed exercise therapy in patients recovering from myocardial infarction. *Psychosomatic Medicine, 6,* 519–527.

Bowman, W. C. (1980). Effects of adrenergic activators and inhibitors on the skeletal muscle. In L. Szekeres (Ed.), *Adrenergic activators and inhibitors*. Berlin: Springer-Verlag.

Breckenridge, A. (1982). Jogger's blocade. *British Medical Journal, 284,* 532–533.

Breslow, L. A., & Enstrom, J. E. (1980). Persistence of health habits and their relationship to mortality. *Preventive Medicine, 9,* 469–483.

Browman, C. P. (1981). Physical activity as a therapy for psychopathology: A reappraisal. *Journal of Sports Medicine and Physical Fitness, 21,* 192–197.

Brown, R. S. (1983). *Assessment of operational mode: A lifestyle test.* Unpublished psychological test, University of Virginia.

Brown, R. S. (1984a). Exercise for stress management in renal dialysis and renal transplantation patients. *Dialysis and Transplantation, 13,* 97–98.

Brown, R. S. (1984b, March). *Long term survivors of cancer.* Paper presented at the Fourth National Conference on Human Values and Cancer, American Cancer Society, New York.

Brown, R. S., Ramirez, D. E., & Taub, J. M. (1978, December). The prescription of exercise for depression. *The Physician and Sportsmedicine, 6,* 34–37, 40–41, 44–45.

Brownell, K. D., Heckerman, C. L., Westlake, R. S., Hayes, S. C., & Monti, P. M. (1978). The effect of couples training and partner cooperativeness in the behavioral treatment of obesity. *Behavior Research and Therapy, 16,* 323–333.

Brownell, K. D., & Stunkard, A. J. (1980). Physical activity in the development and control of obesity. In A. J. Stunkard (Ed.), *Obesity.* Philadelphia: Saunders.

Brownell, K. D., Stunkard, A. J., & Albaum, J. M. (1980). Evaluation and modification of exercise patterns in the natural environment. *American Journal of Psychiatry, 137*(12). 1540–1545.

Bruce, E. H., Frederick, R., Bruce, R. A., & Fisher, L. D. (1976). Comparison of active participants and dropouts in capri cardiopulmonary rehabilitation programs. *American Journal of Cardiology, 37,* 53–60.

Buffone, G. W. (1984). Running and depression. In M. L. Sachs & G. W. Buffone (Eds.), *Running as therapy: An integrated approach.* Lincoln, NE: University of Nebraska Press.

Burgess, S. S. (1976). *Stimulus-Seeking, extraversion, and neuroticism in regular, occasional, and non-exercisers.* Unpublished master's thesis, Florida State University.

Buskirk, E. R., Harris, D., Mendez, J., & Skinner, J. (1971). Comparison of two assessments of physical activity and a survey method for calorie intake. *American Journal of Clinical Nutrition, 24,* 1119–1127.

Byrd, O. E. (1963). Survey of beliefs and practices of psychiatrists on the relief of tension by moderate exercise. *Journal of School Health, 33,* 426–427.

Califano, J. A., Jr. (1979). *Healthy people: The Surgeon General's report on health promotion and disease prevention.* Washington, DC: U.S. Government Printing Office.

Cantwell, J. D., Watt, E. W., & Piper, J. H. (1979). Fitness, aerobic points and coronary risk. *The Physician and Sportsmedicine, 7*(8), 79–84.

Caplan, G. (1964). *Principles of preventative psychiatry.* New York: Basic Books.

Carlsson, C., Dencker, S. J., Grimby, G., & Haggendal, J. (1967). Noradrenaline in human blood plasma and urine during exercise in patients receiving large doses of chlorpromazine. *Acta Pharmacol et Toxicology, 25,* 97–106.

Carlsson, C., Dencker, S. J., Grimby, G., & Haggendal, J. (1968a). Circulatory studies during physical exercise in mentally disordered patients. I. Effects of large doses of chlorpromazine. *Acta Medica Scandinavica, 184,* 499–509.

Carlsson, C., Dencker, S. J., Grimby, G., & Haggendal, J. (1968b). Circulatory studies during physical exercise in mentally disordered patients. II. Effects of physical training with and without administration of chlorpromazine. *Acta Medica Scandinavica, 184,* 511–516.

Carlsson, E., Fellenius, E., Lundborg, P., & Svensson, L. (1978). Beta-adrenoreceptor blockers, plasma potassium, and exercise. *Lancet, ii,* 425–426.

Carmack, M. A., & Martens, R. (1979). Measuring commitment to running: A survey of runners' attitudes and mental states. *Journal of Sport Psychology, 1,* 25–42.

Carmody, T. P., Senner, J. W., Malinow, M. R., & Matarazzo, J. D. (1980). Physical exercise rehabilitation: Long-term dropout rate in cardiac patients. *Journal of Behavioral Medicine, 3,* 163–168.

Carr, D. B., Bullen, B. A., Skrinar, G. S., Arnold, M. A., Rosenblatt, M., Beitens, I. Z., Martin, J. B., & McArthur, J. W. (1981). Physical conditioning facilitates the exercise-induced secretion of beta-endorphin and beta-lipoprotein in women. *The New England Journal of Medicine, 305*(10), 560–563.

Carroll, B. J. (1982). Clinical applications of the dexamethasone suppression test for endogeneous depression. *Pharmakospychiatry, 15,* 19–24.

Carver, C. S. (1979). A cybernetic model of self-attention processes. *Journal of Personality and Social Psychology, 37,* 1251–1281.

Cattell, R. B. (1960). Some psychological correlates of physical fitness and physique. In *Exercise and Fitness* (pp. 138–151). Chicago: The Athletic Institute.

Cattell, R. B., Eber, H. W., & Tatsuoka, M. M. (1970). Handbook for the sixteen personality factor questionnaire (16 PF). Clinical, Educational, Industrial, and Research Psychology. Champaign, IL: Institute for Personality and Ability Testing.

Clarke, H. H. (Ed.). (1973, May). *National adult physical fitness survey.* President's Council on Physical Fitness and Sports Newsletter, special edition.

Colt, E. W. D., Dunner, D. L., Hall, K., & Fieve, R. R. (1981). A high prevalence of affective disorder in runners. In M. H. Sacks & M. L. Sachs (Eds.), *Psychology of running.* Champaign, IL: Human Kinetics Publishers.

Cooper, K. H., Pollock, M. L., Martin, R. P., White, S. R., Linnerude, A. C., & Jackson, A. (1976). Physical fitness levels vs. selected coronary risk factors. *Journal of the American Medical Association, 236,* 166–169.

Cousineau, D., Ferguson, R. J., de Champlain, J., Gauthier, P., Cote, P., & Bourassa, M. (1977). Catecholamines in coronary sinus during exercise in man before and after training. *Journal of Applied Physiology, 43,* 801–806.

Cowen, E. L. (1977). Baby-steps toward primary prevention. *American Journal of Community Psychology, 5,* 1–22.

Cowen, E. L. (1980). The wooing of primary prevention. *American Journal of Community Psychology, 8,* 258–284.

Cowen, E. L., et al. (1975). *New ways in school mental health.* New York: Human Sciences Press.

Crase, D., & Sachs, M. L. (1980). Information retrieval systems for professionals in physical education and sport. *Journal of Physical Education and Recreation, 51*(2), 65–66.

Criqui, M. H., Wallace, R. B., Heiss, G., Mishkel, M., Schonfeld, G., & Jones, G. (1980). Cigarette smoking and plasma high-density lipoprotein cholesterol. Circulation, *62,* (Suppl.), 72–76.

Dahlkoetter, J., Callahan, E. J., & Linton, J. (1979). Obesity and the unbalanced energy equation: Exercise versus eating habit change. *Journal of Consulting and Clinical Psychology, 47,* 898–905.

Daniell, H. B. (1975). Cardiovascular effects of diazepam and chlordiazepozide. *European Journal of Pharmacology, 32,* 58–65.

Danielson, R. R., & Wanzel, R. S. (1978). Exercise objectives of fitness program dropouts. In D. M. Landers and R. W. Christina (Eds.), *Psychology of motor behavior and sport, 1977.* Champaign, IL: Human Kinetics Publishers.

Davison, R. J., & Schwartz, G. E. (1976). The psychobiology of relaxation and related states: A multi-process theory. In D. I. Mostofsky (Ed.), *Behavior control and modification of physiological activity.* Englewood Cliffs, NJ: Prentice-Hall.

Davis, J. F. (1959). *Manual of surface electromyography.* (W. A. D. C. Technical Report 59–184). Montreal, Quebec, Canada: McGill University, Allen Memorial Institute of Psychiatry.

Derogatis, L. R., Lipman, R. S., & Covi, L. (1973). SCL-90: An outpatient psychiatric rating scale (Preliminary report). *Psychopharmacology Bulletin, 9,* 13–27.

deVries, H. A. (1965). Effects of exercise upon residual neuromuscular tension. *Bulletin of the American Association of EMG and Electrodiagnostics, 12,* 12.

deVries, H. A. (1968). Immediate and long term effects of exercise upon resting muscle action potential level. *The Journal of Sports Medicine and Physical Fitness, 8,* 1–11.

deVries, H. A., & Adams, G. M. (1972). Electromyographic comparison of single doses of exercise and meprobamate as to effects on muscular relaxation. *American Journal of Physical Medicine, 51,* 130–141.

deVries, H. A., Burke, R. K., Hopper, T., & Sloan, J. H. (1976). Relationship of resting EMG level to total body metabolism with reference to origin of tissue noise. *American Journal of Physical Medicine, 55,* 139–147.

deVries, H. A., Burke, R. K., Hopper, T., & Sloan, J. H. (1977). Efficacy of EMG biofeedback in relaxation training. *American Journal of Physical Medicine, 56,* 75–81.

deVries, H. A., Simard, C.P., Wiswell, R. A. Heckathorne, E., & Carabetta, V. (1982). Fusimotor system involvement in the tranquilizer effect of exercise. *American Journal of Physical Medicine, 61*(3), 111–122. (Abstract appeared in *Medicine and Science in Sports and Exercise,* 1981, *13*(2), 78.)

deVries, H. A., Wiswell, R. A., Bulbulian, R., & Mortani, T. (1981). Tranquilizer effect of exercise: Acute effects of moderate aerobic exercise on spinal reflex activation level. *American Journal of Physical Medicine, 60,* 57–66.

Dienstbier, R. A. (1984). The effect of exercise on personality. In M. L. Sachs & G. W. Buffone (Eds.), *Running as therapy: An integrated approach.* Lincoln, NE: University of Nebraska Press.

Dienstbier, R. A., Crabbe, J., Johnson, G. O., Thorland, W., Jorgensen, J. A., Sadar, M. M., & Lavelle, D. C. (1981). Exercise and stress tolerance. In M. H. Sacks & M. L. Sachs (Eds.), *Psychology of running.* Champaign, IL: Human Kinetics Publishers.

Dishman, R. K. (1981a). Biologic influences on exercise adherence. *Research Quarterly for Exercise and Sport, 52*(2), 143–159.

Dishman, R. K. (1981b). Prediction of adherence to habitual physical activity. In F. J. Nagle & H. J. Montoye (Eds.), *Exercise in health and disease.* Springfield, IL: Charles C Thomas.

Dishman, R. K. (1981c, May 26). *Psychometric monitoring of training stress during high intensity intermittent exercise.* Paper presented in W. P. Morgan (Chair), Sports Psychology: Psychological Monitoring of Training Stress. Symposium, at the Pan American Sports Medicine Congress, Miami, FL.

Dishman, R. K. (1982a). Compliance/adherence in health-related exercise. *Health Psychology, 1,* 237–267.

Dishman, R.K. (1982b). Health psychology and exercise adherence. *Quest, 33*(2), 166–180.

Dishman, R. K. (1982c). Psychobiologic predictors of exercise behavior. In J. T. Partington, T. Orlick, & J. H. Salmela (Eds.), *Sport in perspective.* Ottawa, Ontario, Canada: The Coaching Association of Canada.

Dishman, R. K. (1983). Predicting exercise compliance using psychometric and behavioral measures of commitment (Abstract). *Medicine and Science in Sports and Exercise, 15*(2), 118.

Dishman, R. K. (1984). Motivation and exercise adherence. In J. M. Silva, III & R. S. Weinberg (Eds.), *Psychological foundations of sport.* Champaign, IL: Human Kinetics Publishers.

Dishman, R. K. (1985). Medical psychology in exercise and sport. *Medical Clinics of North America, 69,* 123–143.

Dishman, R. K., & Gettman, L. R. (1980). Psychobiologic influences on exercise adherence. *Journal of Sport Psychology, 2,* 295–310.

Dishman, R. K., & Gettman, L. R. (1981). Psychological vigor and self-perceptions of increased strength (Abstract). *Medicine and Science in Sports and Exercise, 13*(2), 73.

Dishman, R. K., & Ickes, W. (1981). Self-motivation and adherence to therapeutic exercise. *Journal of Behavioral Medicine, 4*(4), 421–438.

Dishman, R. K., Ickes, W., & Morgan, W. P. (1980). Self-motivation and adherence to habitual physical activity. *Journal of Applied Social Psychology, 10,* 115–132.

Doyne, E. J., Chambless, D. L., & Beutler, L. E. (1983). Aerobic exercise as a treatment for depression in women. *Behavior Therapy, 14,* 434–440.

Edwards, K. R., & Jones, M. R. (1970). Personality changes related to pregnancy and obstetric complications. *Proceedings of the 78th Annual Convention of the American Psychological Association* (341–342).

Eischens, R. R., & Greist, J. H. (1984). Beginning and continuing running: Steps to psychological well-being. In M. L. Sachs & G. W. Buffone (Eds.), *Running as therapy: An integrated approach.* Lincoln, NE: University of Nebraska Press.

Eischens, R. R., Kane, P. M., Wilcox, J. M., & Greist, J. H. (1979). Five easy steps for exercise regimen compliance: A new precise guide to running. *Behavioral Medicine,* 14–17.

Epstein, L. H., & Wing, R. R. (1980). Behavioral approaches to exercise habits and athletic performance. In J. Ferguson & C. B. Taylor (Eds.), *Advances in behavioral medicine.* Holliswood, NY: Spectrum.

Epstein, L. H., Wing, R. R., Koeske, R., Ossip, D., & Beck, S. (1983). A comparison of lifestyle change and programmed aerobic exercise on weight and fitness changes in children. *Behavior Therapy, 13,* 651–665.

Epstein, L. H., Wing, R. R., Thompson, J. K., & Griffiths, M. (1980). Attendance and fitness in aerobics exercise: The effects of contract and lottery procedures. *Behavior Modification, 4,* 465–479.

Epstein, S. E., Robinson, B. F., Kahler, R. L., & Braunwald, E. (1965). Effects of beta adrenergic blocade and the cardiac response to maximal and submaximal exercise in man. *Journal of Clinical Investigation, 44,* 1745.

Epstein, Y., Keren, G., Udassin, R., & Shapiro, Y. (1981). Way of life as a determinant of physical fitness. *European Journal of Applied Physiology, 47,* 1-5.

Erdman, R. A., & Duivenvoorden, H. J. (1983). Psychologic evaluation of a cardiac rehabilitation program: A randomized clinical trial in patients with myocardial infarction. *Journal of Cardiac Rehabilitation, 3,* 696-704.

Eysenck, H. J. (1972). Primaries or second order factors: A critical consideration of Cattell's 16 PF battery. *British Journal of Social and Clinical Psychology, 11,* 265-269.

Eysenck, H. J. (1975). The measurement of emotion: Psychological parameters and methods. In L. Levi (Ed.), *Emotions—their parameters and measurement.* New York: Raven Press.

Eysenck, H. J., Nias, D. K. B., & Cox, D. N. (1982). Sport and personality. In S. Rachman & T. Wilson (Eds.), *Advances in behaviour research and therapy.* Oxford: Pergamon Press.

Fagan, R. M. (1976). Exercise, play and physical training in animals. In P. P. G. Bateson & P. H. Klopfer (Eds.), *Perspectives in ethology* (Vol. 2). New York: Plenum Press.

Farina, A., Fisher, J. D., Getter, H., & Fischer, E. H. (1978). Some consequences of changing people's views regarding the nature of mental illness. *Journal of Abnormal Psychology, 87,* 272-279.

Farmer, P. K., Olewine, D. A., Comer, D. W., Edwards, M. E., Coleman, T. M., Thomas, G., & Hames, C. G. (1978). Frontalis muscle tension and occipital alpha production in young males with coronary prone (type A) and coronary resistant (type B) behavior patterns: Effects of exercise. *Medicine and Science in Sports, 10,* 51.

Farrell, P. A., Gates, W. K., Maksud, M. G., & Morgan, W. P. (1982). Increase in plasma beta-endorphin/beta-lipotropin immunoreactivity after treadmill running in humans. *Journal of Applied Physiology, 52,* 1245-1249.

Fielding, J. E. (1982). Effectiveness of employee health improvement programs. *Journal of Occupational Medicine, 24,* 907-916.

Fitness Ontario. (1981). *Low active adults, who they are, how to reach them.* (A Research Report from the Ministry of Culture and Recreation, Sports and Fitness Branch), Government of Ontario, Toronto, Ontario, Canada.

Fitness Ontario. (1982). *The relationship between physical activity and other health-related lifestyle behaviors.* (A Research Report from the Ministry of Culture and Recreation, Sports and Fitness Branch), Government of Ontario, Toronto, Ontario, Canada.

Flynn, M. G., Mitchell, J. B. and Goldfarb, A. H. (1985). Serum beta-endorphin at two different exercise intensities and the relationship to depression. Paper presented at the *Annual Meeting of the American College of Sports Medicine.* Nashville, Tennessee.

Folkins, C. H., Lynch, S., & Gardner, M. M. (1972). Psychological fitness as a function of physical fitness. *Archives of Physical Medicine and Rehabilitation, 53,* 503-508.

Folkins, C. H., & Sime, W. E. (1981). Physical fitness training and mental health. *American Psychologist, 36,* 373-389.

Frankel, H. M., Stevens, V. J., Dyer, J. R., & Craddick, S. (1983, November 14). *Predictors of change by seniors in a fat-loss program.* Paper presented at the annual meeting of the American Public Health Association, Dallas.

Frankenhaeuser, M. (1970). Catecholamines and behavior. *Brain Research, 24,* 552–553.

Franklin, B. (1984). Exercise program compliance: Improvement strategies: In J. Storbic, H. Jordan, & D. Wilson (Eds.), *Obesity: Practical approaches to treatment.*

Freedson, P. S., Mihevic, P. M., Loucks, A. B., & Girandola, R. N. (1983, May). Physique, body composition and psychological characteristics of competitive female body builders. *The Physician and Sportsmedicine, 11,* 85–93.

Fremont, J. (1983). *The separate and combined effects of cognitively based counseling aerobic exercise for the treatment of mild and moderate depression.* Unpublished doctoral dissertation, The Pennsylvania State University.

Friedlander, W. (1981). The effect of physical exercise on brain physiology and chemistry. In S. Fuenning, K. Rose, F. Strider, & W. Sime (Eds.), *Physical fitness and mental health.* Lincoln, NE: University of Nebraska Foundation.

Gale, J. B., Eckhoff, W. T., & Mogel, S. F. (1984). Factors related to adherence to an exercise program for healthy adults. *Medicine and Science in Sports and Exercise, 16.*

Gallup, G. (1977, October 6). All out fitness craze. *San Francisco Chronicle,* p. 36.

Geller, E. S. (1983). Rewarding safety belt usage at an industrial setting: Tests of treatment generality and response maintenance. *Journal of Applied Behavior Analysis, 16,* 189–202.

Geller, E. S., Johnson, R. P., & Pelton, S. L. (1982). Community-based interventions for encouraging safety belt use. *American Journal of Community Psychology, 10,* 183–195.

Geller, E. S., Mann, M., & Brasted, W. (1977). *Trash can design: A determinant of litter-related behavior.* Paper presented at the meeting of the American Psychological Association, San Francisco.

Geller, E. S. Paterson, L., & Talbott, E. (1982). A behavioral analysis of incentive prompts for motivating seat belt usage. *Journal of Applied Behavior Analysis, 15,* 403–414.

Gellhorn, E. (1958). The physiologic basis of neuromuscular relaxation. *American Medical Association Archives of Internal Medicine, 102,* 392–399.

Gellhorn, E., & Loofbourrow, G. N. (1963). *Emotions and emotional disorders: A neurophysiological study.* New York: Harper & Row.

Gentry, W. D. (1980, May). *Personality predictors of compliance among post-myocardial infarction patients.* Paper presented at the annual meeting of the American College of Sports Medicine, Las Vegas, NV.

George Gallup Organization (1984). *American Health Magazine Survey.* New York, NY.

Gettman, L. R., Pollock, M. L., & Ward, A. (1983, October). Adherence to unsupervised exercise. *The Physician and Sportsmedicine, 11,* 56–66.

Gettman, L. R., Ward, P., & Hagan, R. D. (1982). A comparison of combined running and weight training. *Medicine and Science in Sports and Exercise, 14,* 229–234.

Gibbons, L. W., Blair, S. N., Cooper, K. H., & Smith, M. (1983). Association between coronary heart disease risk factors and physical fitness. *Circulation, 67,* 977–983.

Ginzel, K. H., & Eldred, E. (1970). A possible physiological role for the depression of somatic motor function by reflexes from the cardiopulmonary region. *Proceedings of the Western Pharmaceutical Society, 13,* 188–191.

Glassman, A. H., & Bigger, J. T. (1981). Cardiovascular effects of therapeutic doses of tricyclic antidepressants: A review. *Archives of General Psychiatry, 38,* 815–820.

Goldberg, A. P., Hagberg, J., Delmez, J. A., Carney, R. M., McKevitt, P. M., Ehsani, A. A., & Harter, H. R. (1980). The metabolic and psychological effects of exercise training in hemodialysis patients. *American Journal of Clinical Nutrition, 33,* 1620–1628.

Goldman, H. H., & Goldston, S. E. (Eds.). (1985). *Preventing stress-related psychiatric disorders.* (DHHS Publication No. ADM 85-1366). Washington, DC: U.S. Government Printing Office.

Goldston, S. E. (1977). An overview of primary prevention programming. In D. C. Klein & S. E. Goldston (Eds.), *Primary prevention: An idea whose time has come.* (DHEW Publication No. ADM 77-447). Washington, DC: U.S. Government Printing Office.

Gooch, A. S., Natarajan, G., & Goldberg, H. (1974). Influence of exercise on arrythmias induced by digitalis—diuretic therapy in patients with atrial fibrillation. *American Journal of Cardiology, 33,* 230–237.

Gordon, E., Savin, W., Haskell, W. L., & Bristow, M. (1983). B-andrenergic receptor response to exercise training in the presence of B-1 selective and non-selective blockade. *Circulation, 68,* 148.

Gorsuch, R. L., & Cattell, R. B. (1967). Second-stratum personality factors defined in the questionnaire realm of the 16 PF. *Multivariate Behavioral Research, 2,* 211–214.

Gorsuch, R. L., & Key, M. K. (1974). Abnormalities of pregnancy as a function of anxiety and life stress. *Psychosomatic Medicine, 36,* 352–362.

Gould, D., Weiss, M., & Weinberg, R. S. (1981). Psychological characteristics of successful and nonsuccessful big ten wrestlers. *Journal of Sport Psychology, 3,* 69–81.

Greist, J. H., Klein, M. H., Eischens, R. R., & Faris, J. T. (1978, December). Running out of depression. *The Physician and Sportsmedicine, 6*(12), 49–51; 54; 56.

Greist, J. H., Klein, M. H., Eischens, R. R., & Faris, J. W. (1978, June). Antidepressant running: Running as a treatment for non-psychotic depression. *Behavioral Medicine,* 19–24.

Greist, J. H., Klein, M. H., Eischens, R. R., Faris, J., Gurman, A. S., & Morgan, W. P. (1979). Running as treatment for depression. *Comprehensive Psychiatry, 20,* 41–54.

Groos, K. (1898). *The play of animals.* New York: Appleton.

Gwinup, G. (1975). Effect of exercise alone on the weight of obese women. *Archives of Internal Medicine, 135,* 676–680.

Hamburg, D. A. (1981). *An outlook on stress research and health.* Research on stress and human health, Institute of Medicine Publication 81-05 (pp. xi–xxi).

Hamburg, D. A. Elliott, G. R., & Paron, D. L. (1982). *Health and behavior, frontiers of research in the behavioral sciences.* Washington, DC: National Academy Press.

Hanson, D. L., Van Huss, W., & Strautneik, G. (1967). Effects of forced exercise upon the amount and intensity of the spontaneous activity of young rats. *Research Quarterly, 37,* 221–230.

Hanson, D. S. (1970/1971). The effect of a concentrated program in movement behavior on the affective behavior of four year old children at university elementary school. (Unpublished doctoral dissertation, University of California, Los Angeles) *Dissertation Abstracts International, 31,* 3319A. (University Microfilms No. 71-00629).

Hanson, M. G. (1977/1979). Coronary heart disease, exercise and motivation in middle-aged males. Doctoral dissertation, University of Wisconsin, Madison, Wisconsin. *Dissertation Abstracts International, 37,* 2755B.

Harris, D. V. (1970). Physical activity history and attitudes of middle-aged men. *Medicine and Science in Sports, 2,* 203–208.

Harris, D. V. (1973). *Involvement in sport: A somatopsychic rationale for physical activity.* Philadelphia: Lea & Febiger.

Harris, L. (1978). *Perrier study: "Fitness in America."* Vital and Health Statistics of the National Center for Health Statistics.

Hartley, L. H., Mason, J. W., Hogan, R. P., Jones, L. G., Kotchen, T. A., Mougey, E. H., Wherry, F. E., Pennington, L. L., & Ricketts, P. T. (1972a). Multiple hormonal responses to graded exercise in relation to physical training. *Journal of Applied Physiology, 33,* 602–606.

Hartley, L. H., Mason, J. W., Hogan, R. P., Jones, L. G., Kotchen, T. A., Mougey, E. H., Wherry, F. E., Pennington, L. L., & Ricketts, P. T. (1972b). Multiple hormonal responses to prolonged exercise in relation to physical training. *Journal of Applied Physiology, 33,* 607–610.

Hartz, G. W. (1982). The effect of aerobic conditioning upon mood in clinically depressed men and women. (Unpublished doctoral dissertation, Fuller Theological Seminary—School of Psychology). *Dissertation Abstracts International, 43*(6), 1982-B.

Haskell, W. L. (1979). Mechanisms by which physical activity may enhance the clinical status of cardiac patients. In M. L. Pollock & D. H. Schmidt (Eds.), *Heart disease and rehabilitation.* Boston: Houghton Mifflin.

Hayes, K. J. (1960). Wave analysis of tissue noise and muscle action potentials. *Journal of Applied Physiology, 15,* 749–752.

Haynes, R. B., Taylor, D. W., & Sackett, D. L. (1979). *Compliance in health care.* Baltimore, MD: Johns Hopkins University Press.

Heaman, G., Martinez, J. B., & Polonsky de Pantolini, S. (1970). Psychological aspects of the insulin-dependent diabetic. *Excepta Medica Foundation, 209,* 1980.

Heinzelmann, F., & Bagley, R. W. (1970). Response to physical activity programs and their effects on health behavior. *Public Health Reports, 85,* 905–911.

Hess-Homeier, M. J. (1981). A comparison of Beck's cognitive therapy and jogging as treatments for depression. (Unpublished doctoral dissertation, University of Montana). *Dissertation Abstracts International, 42*(3), 1175-B.

Highlen, P. S., & Bennett, B. B. (1984). Elite divers and wrestlers: A comparison between open- and closed-skill athletes. *Journal of Sport Psychology, 5,* 390–409.

Ho, P., Graham, L., Blair, S., Wood, P., Haskell, W., Williams, P., Terry, R., & Farquhar, J. (1981, August). *Adherence prediction and psychological changes following a one-year randomized exercise program.* Paper presented at the annual meeting of the American Psychological Association, Los Angeles.

Ho, P., Graham, L., Blair, S., Wood, P., Haskell, W., Williams, P., Terry, R., & Farquhar, J. (1981, May 24). *Adherence prediction and psychological/behavioral changes following one-year randomized exercise programs.* Abstracts, Pan American Congress and International Course on Sports Medicine and Exercise Science, Miami, FL, p. 9.

Hollozy, J. O. (1983). Exercise, health, and aging: A need for more information. *Medicine and Science in Sports and Exercise, 15,* 1–5.

Holm, H. J. (1984). 82 agoraphobic married female patients: A follow-up study. *Fokus pa Familien* (Journal for Family Therapy), *12,* 31–49.

Hoyt, M. F., & Janis, I. L. (1975). Increasing adherence to a stressful decision via a motivational balance-sheet procedure: A field experiment. *Journal of Personality and Social Psychology, 31,* 833–839.

Hughes, J. R. (1984). Psychological effects of habitual aerobic exercise: A critical review. *Preventive Medicine, 13,* 66–78.

Humphrey, L. L. (1984). Children's self-control in relation to perceived social environment. *Journal of Personality and Social Psychology, 46,* 178–188.

Ilmarinen, J., & Fardy, P. S. (1977). Physical activity intervention for males with high risk of coronary heart disease: A three-year follow-up. *Preventive Medicine, 6,* 416–425.

Ingjer, F., & Dahl, H. A. (1979). Dropouts from an endurance training program. *Scandinavian Journal of Sports Sciences, 1,* 20–22.

Ismail, A. H., & Sothmann, M. S. (1983). Discrimination power and catecholamine-related variables to differentiate between high and low fit adults. In F. Landry et al. (Eds.), *Health estimation, risk reduction and health promotion, proceedings of the society of prospective medicine* (pp. 129–136).

Ismail, A. H., & Young, R. J. (1973). The effect of chronic exercise on the personality of middle-aged men by univariate and multivariate approaches. *Journal of Human Ergology, 2,* 45–54.

Ismail, A. H., & Young, R. J. (1976). Influence of physical fitness on second and third order personality factors using orthogonal and oblique rotation. *Journal of Clinical Psychology, 32,* 268–272.

Ismail, A. H., & Young, R. J. (1977a). Effect of chronic exercise on the multivariate relationships between selected biochemical and personality variables. *Multivariate Behavioral Research, 12,* 49–67.

Ismail, A. H., & Young, R. J. (1977b). Effect of chronic exercise on the personality of adults. *Annals of the New York Academy of Sciences, 301,* 958–969.

Jacobson, E. (1936). The course of relaxation in muscles of athletes. *American Journal of Psychology, 48,* 98–108.

Jacobson, E. (1938). *Progressive relaxation.* Chicago: University of Chicago.

Janis, I. L., & Mann, L. (1977). *Decision making.* New York: Free Press.

Jason, L. A., & Glenwick, D. S. (1980). An overview of behavioral community psychology. In D. Glenwick & L. Jason (Eds.), *Behavioral community psychology: Progress and prospects.* New York: Praeger.

Jefferson, J. W. (1974). Beta-adrenergic receptor blocking drugs in psychiatry. *Archives of General Psychiatry, 31,* 681–691.

Jefferson, J. W. (1975). A review of the cardiovascular effects and toxicity of tricyclic antidepressants. *Psychosomatic Medicine, 37,* 160–179.

Jenkins, C. D., Hames, C. G., Zyzanski, S. J., Rosenman, R. H., & Friedman, M. (1969). Psychological traits and serum lipids. *Psychosomatic Medicine, 31,* 115–128.

Jette, M. (1971). A blood serum and personality trait profile of habitual exercisers.

Proceedings of the joint meeting of the Canadian Association of Sports Sciences and the American College of Sports Medicine, Toronto, Ontario, Canada.

Johnson, D. T., & Spielberger, C. D. (1968). The effects of relaxation training and the passage of time on measures of state- and trait-anxiety. *Journal of Clinical Psychology, 24,* 20–23.

Johnston-O'Connor, E. J., & Kirschenbaum, D. S. (in press). *Something succeeds like success: Positive self-monitoring for unskilled golfers.* Cognitive Therapy and Research.

Kahn, J. (1973). Who wants safer cars? *World Magazine, 3,* 25–28.

Kanfer, F. H., & Karoly, P. (1972). Self-control: A behavioristic excursion into the lion's den. *Behavior Therapy, 3,* 498–516.

Karbe, W. W. (1966). *The relationship of general anxiety and specific anxiety concerning the learning of swimming.* Unpublished doctoral dissertation, New York University.

Karoly, P. (1977). Behavioral self-management in children: Concepts, methods, issues, and directions. In M. Hersen, R. H. Eisler, & P. M. Miller (Eds.), *Progress in behavior modification* (Vol. 5). New York: Academic Press.

Kau, M. L., & Fisher, J. (1974). Self-modification of exercise behavior. *Journal of Behavior Therapy and Experimental Psychiatry, 5,* 213–214.

Kavanagh, T., Shephard, R. J., Chisholme, A. W., Qureshi, S., & Kennedy, J. (1980). Prognostic indexes for patients with ischemic heart disease enrolled in an exercise-centered rehabilitation program. *American Journal of Cardiology, 44,* 1230–1240.

Kavanagh, T. Shephard, R. J., Doney, H., & Pandit, V. (1973). Intensive exercise in coronary rehabilitation. *Medicine and Science in Sports, 5,* 34–39.

Kavanagh, T., Shephard, R. J., Pandit, V., & Doney, H. (1970). Exercise and hypnotherapy in the rehabilitation of the coronary patient. *Archives of Physical Medicine and Rehabilitation, 51,* 578–587.

Kavanagh, T., Shephard, R. J., & Tuck, J. A. (1975, July). Depression after myocardial infarction. *Canadian Medical Association Journal, 113,* 23–27.

Kavanagh, T., Shephard, R. J., Tuck, J. A., & Qereshi, S. (1977). Depression following myocardial infarction: The effects of distance running. *Annals of the New York Academy of Sciences, 301,* 1029–1038.

Keefe, F. J., & Blumenthal, J. A. (1980). The life fitness program: A behavioral approach to making exercise a habit. *Journal of Behavioral Therapy and Experimental Psychiatry, 11,* 31–34.

Keir, S., & Lauzon, R. (1980). Physical activity in a healthy lifestyle. In P. O. Davidson and S. M. Davidson (Eds.), *Behavioral medicine: Changing health lifestyles.* New York: Brunner/Mazel.

Kendall, P. C., et al. (1978). Cognitive-behavioral and patient education interventions in cardiac catheterization procedures: The Palo Alto Medical Psychology Project. *Journal of Consulting and Clinical Psychology, 47,* 49–58.

Kentala, E. (1972). Physical fitness and feasibility of physical rehabilitation after myocardial infarction in men of working age. *Annals of Clinical Research, 4* (Suppl. 9), 1–84.

King, A. C., & Frederiksen, L. W. (1984). Low-cost strategies for increasing exercise behavior: Relapse prevention training and social support. *Behavior Modification, 8,* 3–21.

Kirschenbaum, D. S. (1984a). Self-regulation and sport psychology: Nurturing an emerging symbiosis. *Journal of Sport Psychology.*

Kirschenbaum, D. S. (1984b). *Self-regulatory failure.* Unpublished manuscript, University of Wisconsin at Madison.

Kirschenbaum, D. S. (in press). *Proximity and specificity of planning and goal-setting: Toward clarification of a conflict in self-regulation.* Unpublished manuscript, University of Wisconsin at Madison.

Kirschenbaum, D. S., & Bale, R. M. (1980). Cognitive-behavioral skills in golf: Brain power golf. In R. M. Suinn (Ed.), *Psychology in sports: Methods and applications.* (pp. 334–343). Minneapolis, MN: Burgess.

Kirschenbaum, D. S., & Flanery, R. C. (1983). Behavioral contracting: Outcomes and elements. In M. Hersen, R. E. Eisler, & P. M. Miller (Eds.), *Progress in behavior modification* (Vol. 15). New York: Academic Press.

Kirschenbaum, D. S., & Flanery, R. C. (in press). *Toward a psychology of behavioral contracting.* Clinical Psychology Review.

Kirschenbaum, D. S., Harris, E. S., & Tomarken, A. J. (1984). Effects of parental involvement in behavioral weight loss therapy for preadolescents. *Behavior Therapy, 15,* 485–500.

Kirschenbaum, D. S., & Karoly, P. (1977). When self-regulation fails: Tests of some preliminary hypotheses. *Journal of Consulting and Clinical Psychology, 45,* 1116–1125.

Kirschenbaum, D. S., Ordman, A. M., Tomarken, A. J., & Holtzbauer, B. (1982). Effects of differential self-monitoring and level of mastery on sports performance: Brain power bowling. *Cognitive Therapy and Research, 6,* 335–342.

Kirschenbaum, D. S., Pedro-Carroll, J. L., & DeVoge, J. B. (1983). A social competence model meets an early intervention program: Description and evaluation of Cincinnati's Social Skills Development Program. In D. F. Ricks & B. S. Dohrenwend (Eds.), *Origins of psychopathology: Problems in research and public policy.* New York: Cambridge University Press.

Kirschenbaum, D. S., & Tomarken, A. J. (1982). On facing the generalization problem: The study of self-regulatory failure. In R. C. Kendall (Ed.), *Advances in cognitive-behavior research and therapy* (Vol. 1, pp. 121–200). New York: Academic Press.

Kirschenbaum, D. S., Tomarken, A. J., & Ordman, A. M. (1982). Specificity of planning and choice applied to self-control. *Journal of Personality and Social Psychology.*

Klerman, G. L., Rounsaville, B., Chevron, E., Neu, C., & Weissman, M. (1979). *Manual for short-term interpersonal psychotherapy (IPT) of depression.* New Haven, CT: Boston Collaborative Depression Project (draft).

Klorman, R., Hilpert, P. L., Michael, R., LaGana, C., & Sveen, O. B. (1980). Effects of coping and mastery modeling on experienced and unexperienced pedodontic patients' disruptiveness. *Behavior Therapy, 11,* 156–168.

Knapp, D., Gutmann, M., Foster, C., & Pollock, M. (1984). Self-motivation among 1984 olympic speedskating hopefuls and emotional response and adherence to training (Abstracts). *Medicine and Science in Sports and Exercise, 16,* 114.

Koch, M. F., & Molnar, G. D. (1974). Psychiatric aspects of patients with unstable diabetes mellitus. *Psychosomatic Medicine, 36.*

Kolata, G. B. (1979a). New drugs and the brain. *Science, 205,* 774–776.

Kolata, G. B. (1979b). Sex hormones and brain development. *Science, 205,* 985–987.

Korol, B., Land, W. J., & Brown, M. J. (1965). Effects of chronic chlorpromazine administration on systemic arterial blood pressure in schizophrenic patients: Relationship of body position to blood pressure. *Clinical Pharmacology Therapy, 6,* 587.

Kostrubala, T. (1981). Running and psychotherapy. In S. I. Fuenning, K. D. Rose, F. D. Strider, and W. E. Sime (Eds.), *Physical fitness and mental health: Proceedings of the research seminar on physical fitness and mental health.* Lincoln, NE: University of Nebraska Foundation.

Kostrubala, T. (1984). Running and therapy. In M. L. Sachs & G. W. Buffone (Eds.), *Running as therapy: An integrated approach.* Lincoln, NE: University of Nebraska Press.

Krestovnikoff, A. (1939). *Fizilogic sports.* Moscow: Fizkultura, Sport.

Kroll, W., & Carlson, R. B. (1967). Discriminant function and hierarchical grouping analysis of karate participants' personality profiles. *Research Quarterly, 38,* 405–411.

Lader, M. (1975). Psychophysiological parameters and methods. In L. Levi (Ed.). *Emotions—Their parameters and measurement.* New York: Raven Press.

LaPorte, R. E., Montoye, H. J., & Caspersen, C. J. (1985). Assessment of physical activity in epidemiologic research: Problems and prospects. *Public Health Reports, 100*(2), 131–146.

Lazarus, R. S. (1966). *Psychological stress and the coping process.* New York: McGraw-Hill.

Lazarus, R. S. (1981). The stress and coping paradigm. In C. Eisdorfer, D. Cohen, A. Kleinman, & P. Maxim (Eds.), *Models of clinical psychopathology* (pp. 177–214). New York: Spectrum.

Lazarus, R. S. (1984). On the primacy of cognition. *American Psychologist, 39,* 124–129.

Ledwidge, B. (1980). Run for your mind: Aerobic exercise as a means of alleviating anxiety and depression. *Canadian Journal of Behavioral Science, 12*(2), 126–140.

Lenfant, C., & Schweizer, (1985). Contributions of health-related biobehavioral research to the prevention of cardiovascular diseases. *American Psychologist, 40,* 217–220.

Leventhal, H., & Cleary, P. (1979). Behavioral modification of risk factors: Technology or science? In M. L. Pollock & D. H. Schmidt (Eds.), *Heart disease and rehabilitation.* Boston: Houghton Mifflin.

Leventhal, H., Safer, M., Cleary, P., & Gutmann, M. (1980). Cardiovascular risk modification by community-based programs for life-style change: Comments on the Stanford study. *Journal of Consulting and Clinical Psychology, 48,* 150–158.

Leventhal, H., Zimmerman, R., & Gutmann, M. (1984). Compliance: A self-regulatory perspective. In D. Gentry (Ed.), *Handbook of behavioral medicine.* New York: Guilford Press.

Lindsay-Reid, E., & Osborn, R. W. (1980). Readiness for exercise adoption. *Social Science and Medicine, 14,* 139–146.

Lindskog, B. D., & Sivarajan, E. S. (1982). A method of evaluation of activity and exercise in a controlled study of early cardiac rehabilitation. *Journal of Cardiac Rehabilitation, 2,* 156–165.

Lindstrom, L., & Broman, H. (1974). *A model describing the power spectrum of myoelectric signals part 11: Summation of motor unit signals* (Technical report 9:74). Research Laboratory in Medicine and Electronics, Goteborg, Sweden.

Lipman, R. S. (1982). Differentiating anxiety and depression in anxiety disorders: Use of rating scales. *Psychopharmacology Bulletin, 18,* 69–77.

Little, J. C. (1969). The athlete's neurosis: A deprivation crisis. *Acta Psychiatrica Scandinavica, 45,* 187–197.

Little, J. C. (1979, March). Neurotic illness in fitness fanatics. *Psychiatric Annals, 9*(3), 49–51; 55–56.

Lobstein, D. D. (1983). *A multivariate study of exercise training effects on beta-endorphin and emotionality in psychologically normal, medically healthy men.* Unpublished doctoral dissertation, Purdue University.

Lobstein, D. D., Mosbacher, B. J., & Ismail, A. H. (1983). Depression as a powerful discriminator between physically active and sedentary middle-aged men. *Journal of Psychosomatic Research, 27,* 69–76.

Locke, E. A., Shaw, K. N., Saari, L. M., & Latham, G. P. (1981). Goal setting and task performance: 1969–1980. *Psychological Bulletin, 90,* 125–152.

Luchins, D. J. (1983). Review of clinical and animal studies comparing the cardiovascular effects of doxepin and other tricyclic antidepressants. *American Journal of Psychiatry, 140,* 1006–1009.

Lundborg, P., Astrom, H., Bengtsson, C., Fellenius, E., von Schenck, H., Svensson, L., & Smith, U. (1981). Effect of beta-adrenoreceptor blocade on exercise performance and metabolism. *Clinical Science, 61,* 299–305.

Mahoney, M. J., & Avener, M. (1977). Psychology of the elite athlete: An exploratory study. *Cognitive Therapy and Research, 1,* 135–141.

Mahoney, M. J., & Thoresen, C. E. (1974). *Self-control: Power to the person.* Monterey, CA: Brooks/Cole.

Malmborg, R., Isaacson, S., & Kallivroussis, G. (1974). The effect of beta blocade and/ or physical training in patients with angina pectoris. *Current Therapy and Research, 16,* 171.

Mandler, G., Mandler, J. M., & Uviller, E. T. (1958). Autonomic feedback, the perception of autonomic activity. *Journal of Abnormal and Social Psychology, 56,* 367–373.

Mann, G. V., Garrett, H. L., Farhi, A., Murray, H., Billings, F. T., Shute, E., & Schwarten, S. E. (1969). Exercise to prevent coronary heart disease. *American Journal of Medicine, 46,* 12–27.

Markoff, R. A., Ryan, P., & Young, T. (1982). Endorphins and mood changes in long-distance running. *Medicine and Science in Sports and Exercise, 14*(1), 11–15.

Marlatt, G. A., & Gordon, J. R. (1980). Determinants of relapse: Implications for the maintenance of behavior change. In P. O. Davidson & S. M. Davidson (Eds.), *Behavioral medicine: Changing health lifestyles* (pp. 410–452). New York: Brunner/Mazel.

Marshall, C. L. (1981). *Toward an educated health consumer: Mass communication and quality in medical care.* (U.S. Public Health Service Pub. No. NIH 77–881). Washington, DC: U.S. Government Printing Office.

Martin, J. E. (1981, April). Exercise management: Shaping and maintaining physical fitness. *Behavioral Medicine Advances, 4,* B-5.

Martin, J. E., & Dubbert, P. M. (1982a). Exercise applications and promotion in behavioral medicine: Current status and future directions. *Journal of Consulting and Clinical Psychology, 50*(6), 1004–1017.

Martin, J. E., & Dubbert, P. M. (1982b). Exercise and health: The adherence problem. *Behavioral Medicine Update, 4,* 17–24.

Martin, J. E., & Dubbert, P. M. (1984). Behavioral management strategies for improving health and fitness. *Journal of Cardiac Rehabilitation, 4,* 200–208.

Martin, J. E., & Dubbert, P. M. (1985). Adherence to exercise. In R. L. Terjung (Ed.), *Exercise and sport sciences review.* New York: MacMillan Company.

Martin, J. E., Dubbert, P. M., Kattell, A. D., Thompson, J. K., Raczynski, J. R., Lake, M., Smith, P. O., Webster, J. S., Sikova, T., & Cohen, R. E. (1984). The behavioral control of exercise in sedentary adults: Studies 1 through 6. *Journal of Consulting and Clinical Psychology, 52,* 795–811.

Martinsen, E. W., Medhus, A., & Sandvik, L. (1984). *The effect of aerobic exercise on depression: A controlled study.* Unpublished manuscript.

Mason, J. W. (1968). A review of psychoendocrine research on the pituitary-adrenal cortical system. *Psychosomatic Medicine, 30,* 576–607.

Mason, J. W., Tolson, W. W., Robinson, J. A., Brady, J. V., Tolliver, G. A., & Johnson, T. A. (1968). Urinary androsterone, eticholanolone, and dyhydroepiaandrosterone responses to 72-hr. avoidance sessions in the monkey. *Psychosomatic Medicine, 30,* 710–720.

Massie, J. F., & Shephard, R. J. (1971). Physiological and psychological effects of training—a comparison of individual and gymnasium programs with a characterization of the exercise "drop-out." *Medicine and Science in Sports, 3,* 110–117.

Matarazzo, J. D. (1982). Behavioral health's challenges to academic, scientific, and professional psychology. *American Psychologist, 37,* 1-14.

McGinnis, J. M. (1985). Recent history of federal initiatives in prevention policy. *American Psychologist, 40,* 205–212.

McIntosh, P. (1980). *"Sport For All" programs throughout the world* (Report prepared for UNESCO, Contract No. 207604). New York: UNESCO.

McNair, D. M., Lorr, M., & Droppleman, L. F. (1971). *Profile of Mood States manual.* San Diego, CA: Educational and Industrial Testing Service.

McPherson, B. D., Paivio, A., Yuhasz, M., Rechnitzer, P., Pickard, H., & Lefcoe, N. (1965). Psychological effects of an exercise program for post-infarct and normal adult men. *Journal of Sports Medicine and Physical Fitness, 8,* 95–102.

Melamed, B. G., & Siegel, L. J. (1975). Reduction of anxiety in children facing hospitalization and surgery by use of filmed modeling. *Journal of Consulting and Clinical Psychology, 43,* 511–521.

Meyer, A. J., Nash, J. D., McAlister, A. L., Maccoby, N., & Farquhar, J. W. (1980). Skills training in a cardiovascular health education campaign. *Journal of Consulting and Clinical Psychology, 48,* 129–142.

Meyers, A. W., Cuvillier, C., Staglgaitis, S., & Cook, C. J. (1980). An evaluation of self-help treatment programs for weight loss. *The Behavior Therapist, 3,* 25–26.

Michael, J. (1980). A placebo-controlled double-blind trial of oxyprenolol versus diazepam in the treatment of anxiety and stress. In P. Kielholz, W. Sigenthaler, P. Taggart, & A. Zanchetti (Eds.), *Psychosomatic cardiovascular disorders—When and how to treat.* Bern: Haus Huber Publishers.

Miller, P. M., Johnson, N. L., Wikoff, R., McMahon, M. F., & Garrett, M. J. (1983).

Attitudes and regimen adherence of myocardial infarction and cardiac bypass patients. *Journal of Cardiac Rehabilitation, 3,* 541–548.

Montoye, H. J. (1975). *Physical activity and health: An epidemiological study of an entire community.* Englewood Cliffs, NJ: Prentice-Hall.

Montoye, H. J., Van Huss, W. D., Olson, H., Pierson, W. R., & Hudec, A. (1957). *Longevity and morbidity of college athletes.* Indianapolis: Phi Epsilon Kappa.

Montoye, H. J., Washburn, R., Servais, S., Ertl, A., Webster, J. G., & Nagle, F. J. (1983). Estimation of energy expenditure by a portable accelerometer. *Medicine and Science in Sports and Exercise, 15,* 403–407.

Morgan, W. P. (1970). Pre-match anxiety in a group of college wrestlers. *International Journal of Sports Psychology, 1,* 7.

Morgan, W. P. (1973a). Influence of acute physical activity on state anxiety. *Proceedings, National College Physical Education Association for Men, 76th Annual Meeting.*

Morgan, W. P. (1973b). Psychological influences on perceived exertion. *Medicine and Science in Sports, 5,* 60–65.

Morgan, W. P. (1977). Involvement in vigorous physical activity with special reference to adherence. *Proceedings of the NCPEAM/NAPECW National Conference,* pp. 235–246.

Morgan, W. P., (1979, February). Negative addiction in runners. *The Physician and Sportsmedicine, 7*(2), 56–63; 67–70.

Morgan, W. P. (1979, March). Anxiety reduction following acute physical activity. *Psychiatric Annals, 9,* 36–45.

Morgan, W. P. (1980a, July). Test of champions: The iceberg profile. *Psychology Today,* 92–99; 101; 108.

Morgan, W. P. (1980b). The trait psychology controversy. *Research Quarterly of Exercise and Sport, 51,* 50–76.

Morgan, W. P. (1981). Psychological benefits of physical activity. In F. J. Nagle & H. J. Montoye (Eds.), *Exercise in health and disease.* Springfield, IL: Charles C Thomas.

Morgan, W. P. (1982). Psychological effects of exercise. *Behavioral Medicine Update, 4,* 25–30.

Morgan, W. P. (1984a). *Coping with mental stress: The potential and limits of exercise intervention* (A state-of-the-art workshop). Final report. Rockville, MD: National Institute of Mental Health.

Morgan, W. P. (1984b). Physical activity and mental health. In H. M. Eckert & H. J. Montoye (Eds.), *Exercise and health.* Champaign, IL: Human Kinetics Publishers.

Morgan, W. P. (1985). Affective beneficence of vigorous physical activity. *Medicine and Science in Sports and Exercise, 17,* 94–100.

Morgan, W. P., & Hammer, W. M. (1974). Influence of competitive wrestling upon state anxiety. *Medicine and Science in Sports, 6,* 58.

Morgan, W. P., Horstman, D.H., Cymerman, A., & Stokes, J. (1980). Exercise as a relaxation technique. *Primary Cardiology, 6,* 48–57.

Morgan, W. P., Horstman, D. H., Cymerman, A., & Stokes, J. (1983). Facilitation of physical performance by means of a cognitive strategy. *Cognitive Therapy and Research, 7,* 251–264.

Morgan, W. P., Montoye, H. J., Brown, D. R., & Johnson, R. W. (1983, April). *Efficacy of the MMPI in predicting health status, health behavior, and quality of life: A 20-year prospective study.* Paper presented at the 18th Annual Symposium on Recent Developments in the Use of the MMPI, Minneapolis, MN.

Morgan, W. P., & Pollock, M. L. (1977). Psychological characterization of the elite distance runner. *Annals of the New York Academy of Sciences, 301,* 382–403.

Morgan, W. P., & Pollock, M. L. (1978). Physical activity and cardiovascular health: Psychological aspects. In F. Landry & W. A. R. Orban (Eds.), *Physical activity and human well-being.* Miami, FL: Symposia Specialists, Inc.

Morgan, W. P., Roberts, J. A., Brand, F. R., & Feinerman, A. D. (1970). Psychological effect of chronic physical activity. *Medicine and Science in Sports, 2,* 213–217.

Morgan, W. P., Roberts, J. A., & Feinerman, A. D. (1971). Psychologic effect of acute physical activity. *Archives of Physical Medicine and Rehabilitation, 52*(9), 422–425.

Morgan, W. P., & Vogel, J. (1976). *Influence of required physical activity on aerobic power, attraction toward physical activity and estimation of physical activity* (Technical report). Natick, MA: U. S. Army Institute of Environmental Medicine.

Morrison, J. K. (1980). The public's current beliefs about mental illness: Serious obstacles to effective community psychology. *American Journal of Community Psychology, 8,* 697–707.

Mountjoy, C. Q., & Roth, M. (1982). Studies in the relationship between depressive disorders and anxiety states. *Journal of Affective Disorders, 4,* 127–161.

Mutrie, N., & Harris, D. V. (1983). *Comparison of moods of students enrolled in jogging and English classes.* Unpublished paper, the Pennsylvania State University.

Neilsen Poll. (1983). Statistical report.

Nideffer, R. M. (1976). Test of attentional and interpersonal style. *Journal of Personality and Social Psychology, 34,* 394–404.

Nidever, J. E. (1959). *A factor analytic study of general muscular tension.* Unpublished doctoral dissertation, University of California at Los Angeles.

Nye, G. R., & Poulsen, W. T. (1974). An activity programme for coronary patients: A review of morbidity, mortality, and adherence after five years. *New Zealand Medical Journal, 79,* 1010–1020.

Oldridge, N. B. (1977a). Compliance of post M.I. patients to exercise programs. *Proceedings, American College of Sports Medicine Conference on Coronary Artery Disease: Prevention, Clinical Assessment, and Rehabilitation.* Oral Roberts University, 99–107.

Oldridge, N. B. (1977b). What to look for in an exercise class leader. *The Physician and Sportsmedicine, 5,* 85–88.

Oldrige, N. B. (1979a, May). Compliance in exercise rehabilitation. *The Physician and Sportsmedicine, 7*(5), 94–98; 101, 103.

Oldridge, N. B. (1979b). Compliance of post-myocardial infarction patients to exercise programs. *Medicine and Science in Sports, 11,* 373–375.

Oldridge, N. B. (1979c). Compliance with exercise programs. In M. L. Pollock & D. H. Schmidt (Eds.), *Heart disease and rehabilitation.* Boston: Houghton Mifflin.

Oldridge, N. B. (1982). Compliance and exercise in primary and secondary prevention of coronary heart disease: A review. *Preventive Medicine, 11,* 56–70.

Oldridge, N. B., Donner, A., Buck, C. W., Jones, N. L., Andrew, G. A., Parker, J. O., Cunningham, D. A., Kavanagh, T., Rechnitzer, P. A., & Sutton, J. R. (1983). Predictive indices for dropout: The Ontario exercise heart collaborative study experience. *American Journal of Cardiology, 51*, 70–74.

Oldridge, N. B. & Jones, N. L. (1983). Improving patient compliance in cardiac rehabilitation: Effects of written agreement and self-monitoring. *Journal of Cardiac Rehabilitation, 3*, 257–262.

Oldridge, N. B., Wicks, J. R., Hanley, R., Sutton, J., & Jones, N. (1978). Noncompliance in an exercise rehabilitation program for men who have suffered a myocardial infarction. *Canadian Medical Association Journal, 118*, 361–364.

Olson, J. M., & Zanna, M. P. (1981, February). *Promoting physical activity: A social psychological perspective.* (Report prepared for the Ontario Ministry of Culture and Recreation). Ontario, Canada.

Olson, J. M., & Zanna, M. P. (1982). *Predicting adherence to a program of physical exercise: An empirical study.* (Report to the Ontario Ministry of Tourism and Recreation). Government of Ontario, Canada.

Osler, W. (1910). The Lumleian lectures on angina pectoris. *The Lancet, 1*, 698.

Paffenbarger, R. S., Wing, A. L., & Hyde, R. T. (1978). Physical activity as an index of heart attack in college alumni. *American Journal of Epidemiology, 108*, 161–175.

Peterson, L., & Ridley-Johnson, R. (1980). Pediatric hospital response to survey on pre-hospital preparation for children. *Journal of Pediatric Psychology, 5*, 1–7.

Peterson, L., & Shigetomi, C. (1981). The use of coping techniques to minimize anxiety in hospitalized children. *Behavior Therapy, 12*, 1–14.

Pitts, F. N., Jr. (1971). Biochemical factors in anxiety neurosis. *Behavioral Science, 16*, 82–91.

Pollock, M. L., Foster, C., Salisbury, R., & Smith, R. (1982). Effects of a YMCA starter fitness program. *The Physician and Sportsmedicine, 10*, 89–102.

Pollock, M. L., Gettman, L. R., Milesis, C. A., Bah, M., Durstine, L., & Johnson, M. (1977). Effects of frequency and duration of training on attrition and incidence of injury. *Medicine and Science in Sports, 9*, 31–36.

Pomerleau, O. (1983). Introduction to the proceedings of the University of Connecticut symposium in employee health and fitness. *Preventive Medicine, 12*, 598–599.

Popejoy, D. I. (1967/1968). The effect of a physical fitness program on selected psychological and physiological measures of anxiety. (Doctoral dissertation, University of Illinois, 1967). *Dissertation Abstracts International, 28*, 4900–4901A.

Powles, A. C. P. (1981). The effects of drugs on the cardiovascular response to exercise. *Medicine and Science in Sports and Exercise, 13*, 252–258.

Raglin, J. S., & Morgan, W. P. (1984). *Influence of acute physical activity and "time-out" (distraction) therapy of blood pressure and state anxiety.* University of Wisconsin.

Rahe, R. H., Rubin, R. T., Gunderson, E. K. E., & Arthur, R. J. (1971). Psychologic correlates of serum cholesterol in man: A longitudinal study. *Psychosomatic Medicine, 33*, 399–401.

Ransford, C. P. (1982). A role for amines in the antidepressant effect of exercise: A review. *Medicine and Science in Sports and Exercise, 14*(1), 1–10.

Rappaport, J. (1977). *Community psychology: Values, research, and action.* New York: Holt, Rinehart & Winston.

Rechnitzer, P. A., Cunningham, D. A., Andrew, G. M., et al. (1983). Relation of exercise to the recurrence rate of myocardial infarction in men. *American Journal of Cardiology, 51,* 65–69.

Redman, J., Armstrong, S., & Ng, K. T. (1983). Free-running activity rhythms in the rat: Entrainment by melatonin. *Science, 219,* 1089–1090.

Reid, E. L., & Morgan, R. W. (1979). Exercise prescription: A clinical trial. *American Journal of Public Health, 69,* 591–595.

Reiff, G., Montoye, H. J., Remington, R. D., Napier, J. A., Metzner, H. L., & Epstein, F. H. (1967). Assessment of physical activity by questionnaire and interview. In M. J. Karvonen & A. J. Barry (Eds.), *Physical activity and the heart* (pp. 336–371). Springfield, IL: Charles C Thomas.

Rejeski, W. J., Morley, D., & Miller, H. S. (1984). The Jenkins activity survey: Exploring its relationship with compliance to exercise prescription and met gain within a cardiac rehabilitation setting. *Journal of Cardiac Rehabilitation, 4,* 90–94.

Reuter, M. A. (1979/1982). *Effect of running on individuals who are clinically depressed.* Unpublished master's thesis, the Pennsylvania State University. (Available from Microform Publications, College of HPER, University of Oregon.)

Reuter, M., Mutrie, N., & Harris, D. V. (1984). *Running as an adjunct to counseling in the treatment of depression.* Unpublished manuscript, the Pennsylvania State University.

Riddle, P. K. (1980). Attitudes, beliefs, behavioral intentions, and behaviors of women and men toward regular jogging. *Research Quarterly for Exercise and Sport, 51,* 663–674.

Risch, S. C., & Pickar, D. (Eds.). (1983). Symposium on endorphins. *Psychological Clinics of North America, 6*(3), 363–521.

Robinson, T. T., & Carron, A. V. (1982). Personal and situational factors associated with dropping out versus maintaining participant in competitive sport. *Journal of Sport Psychology, 4,* 364–378.

Rose, R. M., Gordon, T. P., & Bernstein, I. S. (1972). Plasma testosterone levels in the male rhesus: Influence of sexual and social stimuli. *Science, 178,* 643–645.

Rosen, G. (1958). *A history of public health.* New York: MD Publications.

Roskies, E., Kearney, H., Spevak, M., Surkis, A., Cohen, C., & Gilman, S. (1979). Generalizability and durability of treatment effects in an intervention program for coronary-prone (Type A) managers. *Journal of Behavioral Medicine, 2,* 195–207.

Ryan, A. J. (1983). Exercise is medicine. *The Physician and Sportsmedicine, 11,* 10.

Sable, D. L., Brammell, H. L., Sheehan, M. W., Nies, A. S., Gerber, J., & Horwitz, L. D. (1982). Attenuation of exercise conditioning by beta-adrenergic blocade. *Circulation, 65,* 679–684.

Sachs, M. L. (1978, September). Exercise addiction. *Racing South, 1*(3), 14–16.

Sachs, M. L. (1982). Change agents in the psychology of running. In R. C. Cantu & W. J. Gillespie (Eds.), *Sports medicine, sports science: Bridging the gap.* Lexington, MA: The Collamore Press.

Sacks, M. H., & Sachs, M. L. (Eds.) (1981). *Psychology of running.* Champaign, IL: Human Kinetics Publishers.

Safrit, M. J., Wood, T. M., & Dishman, R. K. (1985). The factorial validity of the physical estimation and attraction scales for adults. *Journal of Sport Psychology, 7,* 166–190.

Salonen, J. T., Puska, R., & Tuomilehto, J. (1982). Physical activity and risk of myocardial infarction, cerebral stroke and death: A longitudinal study in Eastern Finland. *American Journal of Epidemiology, 115,* 526–537.

Sanne, H. M. (1973). Exercise tolerance and physical training of non-selected patients after myocardial infarction. *Acta Medica Scandinavica, 551,* (Suppl.) 1–124.

Sarbin, T. R., & Mancuso, J. C. (1970). Failure of a moral enterprise: Attitudes of the public toward mental illness. *Journal of Consulting and Clinical Psychology, 35,* 159–173.

Schendal, J. (1965). Psychological differences between athletes and non-participants in athletics at three educational levels. *Research Quarterly, 36,* 52–67.

Schildkraut, J. J. (1965). The catecholamine hypothesis of affective disorders: A review of supporting evidence. *American Journal of Psychiatry, 122,* 509–522.

Schwartz, G. E., Davidson, R. J., & Goleman, D. J. (1978). Patterning of cognitive and somatic processes in the self-regulation of anxiety: Effects of meditation versus exercise. *Psychosomatic Medicine, 40,* 321–328.

Seemann, J. C. (1978). *Changes in state anxiety following vigorous exercise.* Unpublished master's thesis, University of Arizona.

Selye, H. (1974). *Stress without distress.* Philadelphia: J. B. Lippincott & Co.

Shapiro, S., Weinblatt, E., & Frank, C. W. (1965). The H.I.P. study of the incidence of myocardial infarction and angina. *Journal of Chronic Diseases, 18,* 527-558.

Shapiro, S., Weinblatt, E., Frank, C., & Sager, R. V. (1969). Incidence of coronary heart disease in a population insured for medical care (HIP). *American Journal of Public health, 59,* 1–101.

Sharkey, B. J. (1979). *Physiology of fitness.* Champaign, IL: Human Kinetics Publishers.

Shephard, R. J. (1978). *Physical activity and aging.* London: Croom Helm.

Shephard, R. J. (1979). Cardiac rehabilitation in prospect. In M. L. Pollock & D. H. Schmidt (Eds.), *Heart disease and rehabilitation.* Boston: Houghton Mifflin.

Shephard, R. J., Corey, P., & Kavanagh, T. (1981). Exercise compliance and the prevention of a recurrence of myocardial infarction. *Medicine and Science in Sports and Exercise, 13,* 1–5.

Shephard, R. J., Morgan, P., Finucane, R., & Schimmelfing, L. (1980). Factors influencing recruitment to an occupational fitness program. *Journal of Occupational Medicine, 22,* 389–398.

Sidney, K. H., & Shephard, R. J. (1976). Attitude toward health and physical activity in the elderly: Effects of a physical training program. *Medicine and Science in Sports, 8,* 246–252.

Sime, W. E. (1971, May). *Post-infarct cardiac rehabilitation.* Paper presented at the annual meeting of the American College of Sports Medicine, Toronto, Ontario, Canada.

Sime, W. E. (1977). A comparison of exercise and meditation in reducing physiological response to stress. (Abstract) *Medicine and Science in Sports, 9,* 55.

Sime, W. E. (1978). Acute relief of emotional stress. *Proceedings of the American Association for the Advancement of Tension Control,* Louisville, Kentucky.

Sime, W. E. (1979a). Psychological concomitants of running. In R. Cox (Ed.), *American Alliance for Health, Physical Education, and Recreation Research Consortium Symposium Papers,* (Vol. 2, Book 2). Washington, DC: American Alliance for Health, Physical Education, and Recreation.

Sime, W. E. (1979b, May). *Ten year follow-up study of exercise adherence in middle aged males.* Paper presented at the annual meeting of the American College of Sports Medicine, Honolulu.

Sime, W. E. (1981). Role of exercise and relaxation in coping with acute emotional stress. In S. I. Fuenning, K. D. Rose, F. D. Strider, and W. E. Sime (Eds.), *Physical fitness and mental health: Proceedings of the research seminar on physical fitness and mental health.* Lincoln, NE: University of Nebraska Foundation.

Sime, W. E., Buell, J. C., & Eliot, R. S. (1980a). Cardiovascular responses to emotional stress (quiz interview) in post-myocardial infarction patients and matched control subjects. *Journal of Human Stress, 6,* 39–46.

Sime, W. E., Buell, J. C., & Eliot, R. S. (1980b). Psychophysiological (emotional) stress testing for assessing coronary risk. *Journal of Cardiovascular and Pulmonary Technique, 8,* 27–31.

Sime, W. E., & Degood, D. E. (1977a). Effective EMG biofeedback and progressive muscle relaxation training on awareness of frontalis muscle tension. *Psychophysiology, 14,* 522–530.

Sime, W. E., & Degood, D. E. (1977b). Stress testing for relaxation training effects. In F. J. McGuigan (Ed.), *Proceedings of the American Association for the Advancement of Tension Control Meeting. (pp. 137–144).* Blacksburg, VA: Universal Publications.

Sime, W. E., Mayes, B., Witte, H., Ganster, D., & Tharp, G. (in press). *Occupational stress testing in the real world.* In F. J. McGuigan, W. E. Sime, & J. Wallace (Eds.), *Stress and tension control* (Vol. II). New York: Plenum Press.

Sime, W. E., Whipple, I., Stamler, J., & Berkson, B. (1978). Variability of heart rate, blood pressure and rate-pressure product response in bicycle and ergometer exercise test in middle age men. In R. Shephard & H. Lavalee (Eds.), *Physical fitness assessment: Principles, practice, and application* (pp. 377–383). Springfield, IL: Charles C Thomas.

Singer, I., & Rotenberg, D. (1973). Mechanisms of lithium action. *New England Journal of Medicine, 289,* 254–260.

Sjoberg, L., & Johnson, T. (1978). Trying to give up smoking: A study of volitional breakdowns. *Addictive Behaviors, 3,* 149–164.

Sjoberg, L., & Samsonowitz, V. (1978). Volitional problems in trying to quit smoking. *Scandinavian Journal of Psychology, 19,* 205–212.

Sloane, R. B., Habits, A., Eveson, M. B., & Payne, R. W. (1961). Some behavioral and other correlates of cholesterol metabolism. *Journal of Psychosomatic Research, 5,* 183–190.

Smith, E. L., & Serfass, R. C. (Eds.). (1981). *Exercise and aging.* Hillside, NJ: Enslow Publishers.

Smith, P. K., & Hagan, T. (1980). Effects of deprivation on exercise play in nursery school children. *Animal Behavior, 28,* 922–928.

Smith, R. E., Smoll, F. L., & Curtis, B. (1979). Coach effectiveness training: A cognitive-behavioral approach to enhancing relationship skills in youth sport coaches. *Journal of Sport Psychology, 1,* 59–75.

Soman, V. R., Veikko, A. K., Deibert, D., Felig, P., & DeFronzo, R. S. (1979). Increased insulin sensitivity and insulin binding to monocytes after physical training. *New England Journal of Medicine, 301,* 200–204.

Sonstroem, R. J. (1978). Physical estimation and attraction scales: Rationale and research. *Medicine and Science in Sports, 10*, 97–102.

Sonstroem, R. J. (1982). Attitudes and beliefs in the prediction of exercise participation. In R. C. Cantu & W. J. Gillespie (Eds.), *Sports medicine, sports science: Bridging the gap.* Lexington, MA: The Collamore Press.

Sonstroem, R. J., & Kampper, K. P. (1980). Prediction of athletic participation in middle school males. *Research Quarterly for Exercise and Sport, 51*, 685–694.

Sonstroem, R. J., & Walker, M. I. (1973). Relationship of attitudes and locus of control to exercise and physical fitness. *Perceptual and Motor Skills, 36*, 1031–1034.

Special Report on Depression Research. (1981). *NIMH Science Reports.* Rockville, MD: National Institutes of Mental Health.

Spielberger, C. D. (1966). Theory and research on anxiety. In C. D. Spielberger (Ed.), *Anxiety and behavior.* New York: Academic Press.

Spielberger, C. D. (Ed.) (1972). *Anxiety: Current trends in theory and research (Vol. 1).* New York: Academic Press.

Spielberger, C. D. (1979). *Understanding stress and anxiety.* London: Harper & Row.

Spielberger, C. D., Gorsuch, R. L., & Lushene, R. (1970). *State-Trait Anxiety Inventory manual.* Palo Alto, CA: Consulting Psychologists Press.

Spielberger, C. D., & Jacobs, G. A. (1978). Stress and anxiety during pregnancy and labor. In L. Zichella & P. Pancheri (Eds.), *Clinical psychoneuroendocrinology in reproduction.* New York: Academic Press.

Spielberger, C. D., & Jacobs, G. A. (1979). Maternal emotions, life stress and obstetric complications. In L. Zichella & P. Pancheri (Eds.), *Psychoneuroendocrinology in reproduction.* Amsterdam, the Netherlands: Elsevier/North Holland Biomedical Press.

Spielberger, C. D., Jacobs, G. A., Russell, S., & Crane, R. S. (1983). Assessment of anger: The State-Trait Anger Scale. In J. N. Buitcher & C. D. Spielberger (Eds.), *Advances in personality assessment (Vol. 2)* (pp. 159–186). Hillsdale, NJ: Lawrence Erlbaum Associates.

Spielberger, C. D., Johnson, E. H., Russell, S. F., Crane, R. S., Jacobs, G. A., & Worden, T. J. (1984). The experience and expression of anger. In M. A. Chesney, S. E. Goldston, & R. H. Rosenman (Eds.), *Anger and hostility in behavioral medicine.* New York: Hemisphere/McGraw Hill.

Spielberger, C. D., & London, P. (1982). Rage boomerangs. *American Health, 1*, 52–56.

Stalonas, P. M., Jr., Johnson, W. G., & Christ, M. (1978). Behavior modification for obesity: The evaluation of exercise, contingency management, and program adherence. *Journal of Consulting and Clinical Psychology, 46*, 463–469.

Stephens, T., Jacobs, D. R., & White, C. C. (1985). A descriptive epidemiology of leisure-time physical activity. *Public Health Reports, 100*(2), 147–158.

Stern, M. J., & Cleary, P. (1982). The national exercise and heart disease project: Long term psychosocial outcome. *Archives of Internal Medicine, 142*, 1093–1097.

Stone, W. (1983, August/September). Predicting who will drop out. *Corporate Fitness and Recreation,* 31–35.

Taylor, C. B., Kraemer, H. L., Bragg, D. A., Miles, L. E., Rule, B., Savia, W. M., & DeBusk, R. F. (1982). A new system for long-term recording and processing of heart rate and physical activity in outpatients. *Computers and Biomedical Research, 16*, 7–17.

Taylor, H. L., Buskirk, E. R., & Remington, R. D. (1973). Exercise in controlled trials of the prevention of coronary heart disease. *Federation Proceedings, 32,* 1623–1627.

Taylor, H. L., Jacobs, D. R., Schucker, B., Knudsen, J., Leon, A. S., & Debacker, G. (1978). A questionnaire for the assessment of leisure time physical activity. *Journal of Chronic Diseases, 31,* 741–755.

Teraslinna, P., Partanen, T., Koskela, A., Partanen, K., & Oja, P. (1969). Characteristics affecting willingness of executives to participate in an activity program aimed at coronary heart disease prevention. *Journal of Sports Medicine and Physical Fitness, 9,* 224–229.

Thaxton, L. (1982). Physiological and psychological effects of short-term exercise addiction on habitual runners. *Journal of Sport Psychology, 4,* 73–80.

Thomas, G. S., Lee, P. R., Franks, P., & Paffenbarger, R. S. (1981). *Exercise and health: The evidence and the implications.* Cambridge, MA: Oelgeschlagen, Gunn & Hain.

Thomas, L. (1977). On the science and technology of medicine. In J. H. Knowles (Ed.), *Doing better and feeling worse: Health in the United States.* New York: Norton.

Thompson, C. E., & Wankel, L. M. (1980). The effects of perceived choice upon frequency of exercise behavior. *Journal of Applied Social Psychology, 10*(5), 436–443.

Thompson, J. K., & Martin, J. E. (1984). Exercise in health modification: Assessment and training guidelines. *The Behavior Therapist, 7*(1), 5–8.

Thoreau, H. D. (1978). In R. Epstein & S. Phillips (Eds.), *The natural man: A Thoreau anthology.* Wheaton, IL: The Theosophical Publishing House.

Tillman, K. (1965). Relationship between physical fitness and selected personality traits. *Research Quarterly, 36,* 483–489.

Tooman, M. E. (1982). *The effect of running and its deprivation on muscle tension, mood, and anxiety.* Unpublished master's thesis, The Pennsylvania State University.

Tu, J., & Rothstein, A. L. (1979). Improvement of jogging performance through application of personality specific motivational techniques. *Research Quarterly, 50,* 97–103.

Turner, J. A. (1983, December 14). Bibliographic data bases help researchers gather information more efficiently. *The Chronicle of Higher Education, 27*(16), 27–28.

Turner, R. D., Pooly, S., & Sherman, A. R. (1976). A behavioral approach to individualized exercise programming. In J. D. Krumboltz & C. E. Thoresen (Eds.)., *Counseling methods.* New York: Holt, Rinehart & Winston.

U. S. Department of Health and Human Services. (1982). *Prevention '82. Public Health Service, Office of Disease Prevention and Health Promotion.* (DHHS (PHS) Publication No. 82-50157). Washington, DC: U.S. Government Printing Office.

Uusitupa, M., Aro, A., & Pietkainen, M. (1980). Severe hypoglycaemia caused by physical strain and pindolol therapy. *Annals of Clinical Research, 12,* 25–27.

Vance, B. (1976). Using contracts to control weight and to improve cardiovascular physical fitness. In J. D. Krumboltz & C. E. Thoresen (Eds.), *Counseling methods.* New York: Holt, Rinehart & Winston.

Vanhees, L., Fagard, R., & Amery, A. (1982). Influence of beta adrenergic blocade on effects of physical training in patients with ischemic heart disease. *British Heart Journal, 48,* 33–38.

Veith, R. C., Raskin, M. A., Caldwell, J. H., et al. (1982). Cardiovascular effects of tricyclic antidepressants in depressed patients with chronic heart disease. *New England Journal of Medicine, 306,* 954–959.

Vohra, J., Burrows, J. D., & Sloman, J. (1975). Assessment of cardiovascular side effects of therapeutic doses of tricyclic antidepressant drugs. *Australian New Zealand Journal of Medicine, 5,* 7–11.

Von Euler, C., & Soderberg, U. (1957). The influence of hypothalmic thermoceptive structures on the electroencephalogram and gamma motor activity. *EEG & Clinical Neurophysiology, 9,* 391–408.

Voss, H. (1971). Tabelle der absoluten und relativen muskelspindelzahlen der menschlichen skelettmuskulatur. *Anat. Anz., 129,* 562–572.

Wallace, R. K., & Benson, H. (1972). The physiology of meditation. *Scientific American, 226,* 85–90.

Wankel, L. M. (1980). Involvement in vigorous physical activity: Considerations for enhancing self-motivation. In R. R. Danielson & K. F. Danielson (Eds.), *Fitness motivation: Proceedings of the Geneva Park Workshop.* Toronto: Orcol Publications.

Wankel, L. M. (in press). Exercise adherence and leisure activity: Patterns of involvement and interventions to facilitate regular activity. In R. K. Dishman (Ed.), *Exercise adherence and public health.* Champaign, IL: Human Kinetics Publishers.

Wankel, L. M., & Graham, J. H. (1984). *The effects of a decision balance-sheet intervention upon exercise adherence of high and low self-motivated females.* Manuscript submitted for publication.

Wankel, L. M., & Thompson, C. (1977). Motivating people to be physically active: Self-persuasion vs. balanced decision making. *Journal of Applied Social Psychology, 7,* 332–340.

Wankel, L. M., & Yardley, J. K. (1982, August). *An investigation of the effectiveness of a structured social support program for increasing exercise adherence of high and low self-motivated adults.* Paper presented at the annual conference of the Canadian Parks and Recreation Association, Saskatoon, Saskatchewan.

Wankel, L. M., Yardley, J. F., & Graham, J. (1985). The effects of motivational interventions upon the exercise adherence of high and low self-motivated adults. *Canadian Journal of Applied Sport Sciences, 10,* 147–156.

Ward, A., & Morgan, W. P. (1984). Adherence patterns of healthy men and women enrolled in an adult exercise program. *Journal of Cardiac Rehabilitation, 4,* 143–152.

Watson, G. S., Zador, P. L., & Wilks, A. (1980). The repeal of helmet use laws and increased motorcyclist mortality in the United States, 1975–1978. *American Journal of Public Health, 70,* 579–585.

Watson, G. S., Zador, P. L., & Wilks, A. (1981). Helmet use, helmet use laws, and motorcyclist fatalities. *American Journal of Public Health, 71,* 297–300.

Weinstein, W. S., & Meyers, A. W. (1983). Running as treatment for depression: Is it worth it? *Journal of Sport Psychology, 5,* 288–301.

Weissberg, R. P., et al. (1981). The effects of social problem solving on the problem-solving skills and adjustment of 3rd grade children. *Journal of Consulting and Clinical Psychology, 49,* 251–260.

Weissman, M. M. (1980). Use of a self-report symptom scale to detect depression in a community sample. *American Journal of Psychiatry, 137,* 1081.

Whalen, R. E., & Simon, N. G. (1984). Biological motivation. *Annual Review of Psychology, 35,* 257–276.

White, J. A., Ismail, A. H., & Bottoms, G. D. (1975). Variability of corticosteroid responses during exercise stress in active and sedentary middle-aged males. *British Journal of Sports Medicine, 9,* 1–8.

Whiting. H. T., & Stembridge, D. E. (1965). Personality and the persistent nonswimmer. *Research Quarterly, 36,* 348–356.

Wilhelmson, L., Sanne, H., Elmfeldt, D., Tibblin, B., Grimby, G., & Wedel, G. (1975). A controlled trial of physical training after myocardial infarction. *Preventive Medicine, 4,* 491–508.

Wilmore, J. H., Constable, S. H., Stanforth, P. R., Tasao, W. Y., Rotkis, T. C., Paicius, R. M., Mattern, C. M., & Ewy, G. A. (1982). Prevalence of coronary heart disease risk factors in 13 to 15 year old boys. *Journal of Cardiac Rehabilitation, 2,* 223–233.

Wilson, V. E., Berger, B. G., & Bird, E. I. (1981). Effects of running and of an exercise class on anxiety. *Perceptual and Motor Skills, 53,* 472–474.

Wood, P. D., Haskell, W. L., Blair, S. N., Williams, P. T., Krauss, R. M., Lindgren, F. T., Alberg, J., Ho, P., & Farquhar, J. W. (1983). Increased exercise level and plasma lipoprotein concentrations: A one-year randomized, controlled study in sedentary, middle-age men. *Metabolism, 32,* 31–39.

Wyke, B. (1982). Receptor systems in lumbrosacral tissues in relation to the production of low back pain. In A. A. White & S. L. Gordon (Eds.). *AAOS symposium on ideopathic low back pain.* St. Louis: C. V. Mosby.

Wysocki, T., Hall, G., Iwata, B., & Riordan, M. (1979). Behavioral management of exercise: Contracting for aerobic points. *Journal of Applied Behavior Analysis, 12,* 55–64.

Yasin, S., Alderson, M. Marv, J. W., et al. (1967). Assessment of habitual physical activity apart from occupation. *British Journal of Preventive and Social Medicine, 21,* 163–169.

Yates, A., Leehey, K., & Shisslak, C. M. (1983, February). Running: An analogue of anorexia? *The New England Journal of Medicine, 308*(5), 251–255.

Young, R. J. (1979). The effect of regular exercise on cognitive functioning and personality. *British Journal of Sports Medicine, 13,* 110-117.

Young, R. J., & Ismail, A. H. (1976a). Personality differences of adult men before and after a physical fitness program. *Research Quarterly, 47,* 513–519.

Young, R. J., & Ismail, A. H. (1976b). Relationship between anthropometric, physiological, biochemical and personality variables before and after a four month conditioning program for middle-aged men. *Journal of Sports Medicine and Physical Fitness, 16,* 267–276.

Young, R. J., & Ismail, A. H. (1977). Comparison of selected physiological and personality variables in regular and nonregular adult male exercisers. *Research Quarterly, 48,* 617–622.

Zajonc, R. B. (1984). On the primacy of affect. *American Psychologist, 39,* 117–123.

Zastowny, T. R., Kirschenbaum, D. S., & Meng, I. (in press). Effects of stress inoculation training on children before, during, and after hospitalization for surgery. *Journal of Consulting and Clinical Psychology.*

Zipp, P. (1978). The effect of electrode parameters on the bandwidth of the surface EMG power-density spectrum. *Medicine and Biology in Engineering and Computing, 16,* 537–541.

Zitrin, C. M., Klein, D. F., & Woerner, M. G. (1978). Behaviour therapy, supportive psychotherapy, imipramine, and phobias. *Archives of General Psychiatry, 35,* 307–316.

Zitrin, C. M., Klein, D. F., & Woerner, M. G. (1980). Treatment of agoraphobia with group exposure in vivo and imipramine. *Archives of General Psychiatry, 37,* 63–72.

INDEX